IMMUNIZATION SAFETY REVIEW

VACCINES AND AUTISM

Immunization Safety Review Committee
Board on Health Promotion and Disease Prevention

INSTITUTE OF MEDICINE
OF THE NATIONAL ACADEMIES

D1089507

THE NATIONAL ACADEMIES PRESS
Washington, D.C.
www.nap.edu

THE NATIONAL ACADEMIES PRESS 500 Fifth Street, N.W. Washington, DC 20001

NOTICE: The project that is the subject of this report was approved by the Governing Board of the National Research Council, whose members are drawn from the councils of the National Academy of Sciences, the National Academy of Engineering, and the Institute of Medicine. The members of the committee responsible for the report were chosen for their special competences and with regard for appropriate balance.

This study was supported by Contract No. N01-OD-4-2139, Task Order #74 between the National Academy of Sciences and Centers for Disease Control and Prevention and the National Institute of Allergy and Infectious Diseases of the National Institutes of Health. Any opinions, findings, conclusions, or recommendations expressed in this publication are those of the author(s) and do not necessarily reflect the view of the organizations or agencies that provided support for this project.

International Standard Book Number 0-309-09237-X (Book)
International Standard Book Number 0-309-53275-2 (PDF)

Additional copies of this report are available from the National Academies Press, 500 Fifth Street, N.W., Lockbox 285, Washington, DC 20055; (800) 624-6242 or (202) 334-3313 (in the Washington metropolitan area); Internet, http://www.nap.edu.

For more information about the Institute of Medicine, visit the IOM home page at: **www.iom.edu.**

The serpent has been a symbol of long life, healing, and knowledge among almost all cultures and religions since the beginning of recorded history. The serpent adopted as a logotype by the Institute of Medicine is a relief carving from ancient Greece, now held by the Staatliche Museen in Berlin.

"Knowing is not enough; we must apply.
Willing is not enough; we must do."
—Goethe

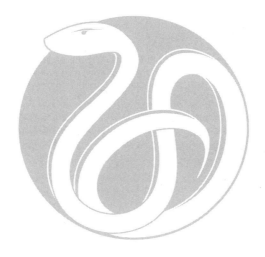

INSTITUTE OF MEDICINE
OF THE NATIONAL ACADEMIES

Adviser to the Nation to Improve Health

THE NATIONAL ACADEMIES
Advisers to the Nation on Science, Engineering, and Medicine

The **National Academy of Sciences** is a private, nonprofit, self-perpetuating society of distinguished scholars engaged in scientific and engineering research, dedicated to the furtherance of science and technology and to their use for the general welfare. Upon the authority of the charter granted to it by the Congress in 1863, the Academy has a mandate that requires it to advise the federal government on scientific and technical matters. Dr. Bruce M. Alberts is president of the National Academy of Sciences.

The **National Academy of Engineering** was established in 1964, under the charter of the National Academy of Sciences, as a parallel organization of outstanding engineers. It is autonomous in its administration and in the selection of its members, sharing with the National Academy of Sciences the responsibility for advising the federal government. The National Academy of Engineering also sponsors engineering programs aimed at meeting national needs, encourages education and research, and recognizes the superior achievements of engineers. Dr. Wm. A. Wulf is president of the National Academy of Engineering.

The **Institute of Medicine** was established in 1970 by the National Academy of Sciences to secure the services of eminent members of appropriate professions in the examination of policy matters pertaining to the health of the public. The Institute acts under the responsibility given to the National Academy of Sciences by its congressional charter to be an adviser to the federal government and, upon its own initiative, to identify issues of medical care, research, and education. Dr. Harvey V. Fineberg is president of the Institute of Medicine.

The **National Research Council** was organized by the National Academy of Sciences in 1916 to associate the broad community of science and technology with the Academy's purposes of furthering knowledge and advising the federal government. Functioning in accordance with general policies determined by the Academy, the Council has become the principal operating agency of both the National Academy of Sciences and the National Academy of Engineering in providing services to the government, the public, and the scientific and engineering communities. The Council is administered jointly by both Academies and the Institute of Medicine. Dr. Bruce M. Alberts and Dr. Wm. A. Wulf are chair and vice chair, respectively, of the National Research Council.

www.national-academies.org

Health Promotion and Disease Prevention Board Liaison

RICHARD B. JOHNSTON, Jr., M.D., Professor of Pediatrics, Associate
Dean for Research Development, University of Colorado School of
Medicine and National Jewish Medical and Research Center, Denver, CO

Study Staff

KATHLEEN STRATTON, Ph.D., Study Director
ALICIA GABLE, M.P.H., Program Officer
DONNA ALMARIO, M.P.H., Research Associate
AMY B. GROSSMAN, Senior Project Assistant
ROSE MARIE MARTINEZ, Sc.D., Director, Board on Health Promotion and
Disease Prevention

Contract Editor

STEVEN J. MARCUS, Ph.D.

Reviewers

This report has been reviewed in draft form by individuals chosen for their diverse perspectives and technical expertise, in accordance with procedures approved by the NRC's Report Review Committee. The purpose of this independent review is to provide candid and critical comments that will assist the institution in making its published report as sound as possible and to ensure that the report meets institutional standards for objectivity, evidence, and responsiveness to the study charge. The review comments and draft manuscript remain confidential to protect the integrity of the deliberative process. We wish to thank the following individuals for their review of this report:

Ann Bostrom, Georgia Institute of Technology
Daniel Crimmins, Westchester Institute for Human Development; New York Medical College
Geraldine Dawson, University of Washington
Bradley Doebbeling, Indiana University-Purdue University Indianapolis, Health Services Research Service
Neal Halsey, Johns Hopkins University
Robin L. Hansen, University of California, Davis; M.I.N.D. Institute
Howard Hu, Harvard University; Brigham and Women's Hospital
Gerald Mandell, University of Virginia Health Center
Peter H. Meyers, George Washington University
Craig Newschaffer, Johns Hopkins University Bloomberg School of Public Health

Richard Rheingans, Emory University, Rollins School of Public Health
Brian Ward, McGill University-Montreal General Hospital
Andrew Zimmerman, Johns Hopkins University

Although the reviewers listed above have provided many constructive comments and suggestions, they were not asked to endorse the conclusions or recommendations nor did they see the final draft of the report before its release. The review of this report was overseen by **Robert S. Lawrence**, Johns Hopkins University, and **Floyd E. Bloom**, Scripps Research Institute. Appointed by the National Research Council and Institute of Medicine, they were responsible for making certain that an independent examination of this report was carried out in accordance with institutional procedures and that all review comments were carefully considered. Responsibility for the final content of this report rests entirely with the authoring committee and the institution.

Foreword

Vaccines are among the greatest public health accomplishments of the past century. In recent years, however, a number of concerns have been raised about both the safety of and the need for certain immunizations. Indeed, immunization safety is a contentious area of public health policy, with discourse around it having become increasingly polarized and exceedingly difficult. The numerous controversies and allegations surrounding immunization safety signify an erosion of public trust in those responsible for vaccine research, development, licensure, scheduling, and policymaking. Because vaccines are so widely used—and because state laws require that children be vaccinated to enter daycare and school, in part to protect others—immunization safety concerns should be vigorously pursued in order to restore this trust.

It is in this context that the Institute of Medicine (IOM) was approached over three years ago by the Centers for Disease Control and Prevention and the National Institutes of Health to convene an independent committee that could provide timely and objective assistance to the Department of Health and Human Services in reviewing emerging immunization safety concerns.

The IOM was chartered by the National Academy of Sciences in 1970 to serve as an adviser to the federal government on issues affecting the public's health, as well as to act independently in identifying important issues of medical care, research, and education. The IOM thus brings to this mission three decades of experience in conducting independent analyses of significant public health policy issues. In particular, as described in more detail in this report, the IOM has a long history of involvement in vaccine safety. The IOM published its first major vaccine safety report in 1977, followed by a subsequent report in 1988; both focused on the safety of polio vaccines. Two subsequent major reports, published in 1991 and 1994, examined the adverse effects of childhood vaccines. Since then, the IOM has conducted several smaller studies and workshops focused on various vaccine safety topics. These studies were well received by both the public and policymakers, and previous IOM committees on vaccine safety issues have been viewed as objective and credible.

Given the sensitive nature of the present immunization safety review study, the IOM felt it was especially critical to establish strict criteria for committee membership. These criteria prevented participation by anyone with financial ties to vaccine manufacturers or their parent companies, or who had given expert testimony on issues of vaccine safety.

The rationale for imposing these stringent criteria was twofold. First, given growing public concern about vaccine safety and the public scrutiny surrounding this committee's work, it was important to establish standards that would preclude any real or perceived conflict of interest or bias on the part of the committee members. No member has any vested interest in any of the vaccine safety questions that will come before the committee. Second, the IOM wanted to ensure that no committee member had participated in the development or evaluation of a vaccine under study.

Thus, the IOM has convened a distinguished panel of 13 members who are experts in a number of pertinent fields, including pediatrics, neurology, immunology, internal medicine, infectious diseases, genetics, epidemiology, biostatistics, risk perception and communication, decision analysis, public health, nursing, and ethics. The committee members were chosen because they are leading authorities in their respective fields, are well respected by their colleagues, and have no conflicts of interest. This committee brought a fresh perspective to these critically important issues and approached its charge with impartiality and scientific rigor.

As with all reports from the IOM, the committee's work was reviewed by an independent panel of experts. The purpose of the review process is to enhance the clarity, cogency, and accuracy of the final report and to ensure that the authors and the IOM are creditably represented by the report published in their names. The report review process is overseen by the National Research Council's (NRC) Report Review Committee (RRC), comprising approximately 30 members of the National Academy of Sciences, National Academy of Engineering, and IOM. A select panel of reviewers with a diverse set of perspectives are asked to critique the report. Unlike the selection criteria for committee membership, many reviewers will have strong opinions and interests related to the report topic. The composition of the review panel is not disclosed to the committee until after the report is approved for release. While the committee must consider and evaluate all comments from reviewers, it is not obligated to change its report in response to the reviewers' comments. The committee must, however, justify its responses to the reviewers' comments to the satisfaction of the RRC's review monitor and the IOM's review coordinator. A report may not be released to the sponsors or the public, nor may its findings be disclosed, until after the review process has been satisfactorily completed and all authors have approved the revised draft.

This report represents the unanimous conclusions and recommendations of that dedicated committee whose members deliberated a critical health issue. I am grateful to the committee and its able staff for their efforts on behalf of the public's health.

Harvey V. Fineberg
President, Institute of Medicine

Acknowledgments

The committee would like to acknowledge the many speakers and attendees at its open meeting held on February 9, 2004, at the National Academy of Sciences building in Washington, DC. The discussions were informative and helpful. The committee would also like to thank those people who submitted information to the committee through the mail or via e-mail. Finally, the committee thanks the IOM staff for their dedication to this project. Without their commitment, attention to detail, creativity, sensitivity, and hard work, this project would be unworkable.

Contents

Executive Summary

ABSTRACT

This eighth and final report of the Immunization Safety Review Committee examines the hypothesis that vaccines, specifically the measles-mumps-rubella (MMR) vaccine and thimerosal-containing vaccines, are causally associated with autism. The committee reviewed the extant published and unpublished epidemiological studies regarding causality and studies of potential biologic mechanisms by which these immunizations might cause autism. The committee concludes that the body of epidemiological evidence favors rejection of a causal relationship between the MMR vaccine and autism. The committee also concludes that the body of epidemiological evidence favors rejection of a causal relationship between thimerosal-containing vaccines and autism. The committee further finds that potential biological mechanisms for vaccine-induced autism that have been generated to date are theoretical only.

The committee does not recommend a policy review of the current schedule and recommendations for the administration of either the MMR vaccine or thimerosal-containing vaccines. The committee recommends a public health response that fully supports an array of vaccine safety activities. In addition, the committee recommends that available funding for autism research be channeled to the most promising areas. The committee makes additional recommendations regarding surveillance and epidemiological research, clinical studies, and communication related to these vaccine safety concerns. Please see Box ES-1 for a summary of all conclusions and recommendations.

Immunization to protect children and adults from infectious diseases is one of the greatest achievements of public health. Immunization is not without risks, however. It is well established, for example, that the oral polio vaccine on rare occasion has caused paralytic polio and that vaccines sometimes produce anaphylactic shock. Given the widespread use of vaccines, state mandates requiring vaccination of children for entry into school, college, or day care, and the importance of ensuring that trust in immunization programs is justified, it is essential that safety concerns receive assiduous attention.

At the request of the sponsoring agencies, the Centers for Disease Control and Prevention (CDC) and the National Institutes of Health (NIH), the Institute of Medicine (IOM) established the Immunization Safety Review Committee to evaluate the evidence on possible causal associations between immunizations and certain adverse outcomes, and to then present conclusions and recommendations. The committee's mandate also includes assessing the broader significance for society of these immunization safety issues.

The specific vaccine safety hypotheses issues examined by the committee are determined by the Interagency Vaccine Group (IAVG), whose members represent several units of the Department of Health and Human Services: the CDC's National Vaccine Program Office, National Immunization Program, and National Center for Infectious Diseases; the NIH's National Institute of Allergy and Infectious Diseases; the Food and Drug Administration (FDA); the Health Resources and Services Administration's National Vaccine Injury Compensation Program; and the Centers for Medicare & Medicaid Services. The IAVG also includes representation from the Department of Defense and the Agency for International Development. The committee has issued seven previous reports on vaccine safety issues over the three-year study period (2001-2003). This eighth and final report from the committee examines the hypothesis that vaccines, specifically the measles-mumps-rubella (MMR) vaccine and vaccines containing the preservative thimerosal, cause autism. In its first two reports that were published in 2001, the committee examined the hypothesized causal association between the MMR vaccine and autism, and thimerosal-containing vaccines and neurodevelopmental disorders, respectively (IOM, 2001a,b). The IAVG asked the committee to revisit the hypothesized causal association between vaccines and autism in its final report in order to update its conclusions and recommendations based on the significant number of studies that have been undertaken in the last three years.

The committee begins from a position of neutrality regarding the specific immunization safety hypothesis under review. That is, there is no presumption that a specific vaccine (or vaccine component) does or does not cause the adverse event in question. The weight of the available clinical and epidemiologic evidence determines whether it is possible to shift from that neutral position to a finding for causality ("the evidence favors acceptance of a causal relationship") or against causality ("the evidence favors rejection of a causal relationship"). The committee does not conclude that the vaccine does not cause the adverse event merely because the evidence is inadequate to support causality. Instead, it maintains a neutral position, concluding that the "evidence is inadequate to accept or reject a causal relationship."

The committee's causality assessments must be guided by an understanding of relevant biological processes. Therefore the committee's scientific assessment includes consideration of biological mechanisms by which immunizations might cause an adverse event. The examination of experimental evidence for biological mechanisms has been referred to in previous reports of this committee (IOM, 2001a,b) and others (IOM, 1991, 1994) as an assessment of "biological plausibility." The committee has noted, however, that the term "biologic plausibility" is a source of confusion on at least two fronts. First, it is associated with a particular set of guidelines (sometimes referred to as the Bradford Hill criteria) for causal inference from epidemiological evidence (Hill, 1965); second, readers sometimes regard the term with a degree of certainty or precision the committee never intended. For example, a relationship between immunization and a particular adverse event may be found to be biologically plausible at the same time that the epidemiological evidence is found to be inadequate to accept or reject a causal relationship.

Given the resulting lack of clarity, the committee adopted a new terminology and a new approach to its discussions of experimental biological data in its third report (IOM, 2002). The committee now reviews evidence regarding "biological *mechanisms*" that might be consistent with the proposed relationship between immunization and a given adverse event.

The biological mechanism evidence reviewed in this report comes from human, animal, and *in vitro* studies of biological or pathophysiological processes. If the committee identifies evidence of biological mechanisms that could be operating, it offers a summary judgment of that body of evidence as weak, moderate, or strong. Although the committee tends to judge biological evidence in humans as "stronger" than biological evidence from highly contrived animal models or *in vitro* systems, the summary judgment of the strength of the evidence also depends on the quantity (e.g., number of studies or number of subjects in a study) and quality (e.g., the nature of the experimental system or study design) of the evidence. Obviously, the conclusions drawn from this review depend both on the specific data and scientific judgment. To ensure that its own summary judgment is defensible, the committee aims to be as explicit as possible regarding the strengths and limitations of the biological data.

In this report, the committee examines the hypothesis of whether the MMR vaccine and the use of vaccines containing the preservative thimerosal can cause autism. Autism is a complex and severe set of developmental disorders characterized by sustained impairments in social interaction, impairments in verbal and nonverbal communication, and stereotypically restricted or repetitive patterns of behaviors and interests (APA, 1994; Filipek et al., 1999; Volkmar and Pauls, 2003). Over time, research has identified subtle differences in the onset and progression of autistic symptoms. Autism is classified under the umbrella category of "pervasive developmental disorders" (PDDs) (APA, 2000). PDD refers to a continuum of related cognitive and neurobehavioral disorders that reflects the heterogeneity of symptoms and clinical presentations, and includes autistic disorder, childhood disintegrative disorder, Asperger's syndrome, Rett's syndrome, and pervasive developmental disorder not otherwise specified (PDD-NOS, or atypical autism). The term "autistic spectrum disorders" (ASD) has come into common use and is essentially synonymous with the term PDD (Volkmar et al., 2003). In this report, the terms "autism," "autistic," and "autistic spectrum disorders" are used interchangeably to refer to this broader group of pervasive developmental disorders.[1] Although Rett's syndrome is among the autistic spectrum disorders, it is considered by many to be a distinct neurologic disorder and thus its diagnosis is not included in most research that has evaluated the association of the vaccines and autism.

There is considerable uncertainty about the prevalence and incidence of autism and trends over time. Some studies have found an increase, but it is difficult to discern how much of the observed increase is real or possibly due to other factors, such as the adoption of a broader diagnostic concept of autism, improved recognition of autism, or variations in the precision of the studies (Fombonne, 1999, 2003; Gillberg and Wing, 1999).

In the committee's first report, which reviewed the hypothesized causal association between the MMR vaccine and autism (IOM, 2001a), the committee concluded that the evidence at the time favored rejection of a causal relationship at the population level between MMR vaccine and autism. The committee's conclusion did not exclude the possibility that MMR could contribute to autism in a small number of children because the epidemiological studies lacked sufficient precision to assess rare occurrences; it was possible, for example, that epidemiological studies would not detect a relationship between autism and MMR vaccination in a subset of the population with a genetic predisposition to autism. The biological models for an association between MMR and autism were not established but nevertheless not disproved.

In a subsequent report, the committee reviewed the hypothesized link between thimerosal-containing vaccines (TCVs) and a broad range of neurodevelopmental disorders (NDD), including autism (IOM, 2001b). Thimerosal, an organic mercury compound, has been used as a preservative in some vaccines and other biological and pharmaceutical products since the 1930s. FDA regulations require the use of preservatives in multidose vials of vaccines, except live virus vaccines, to prevent fungal and bacterial contamination (General Biologics Product Stan-

---

[1]The term "autistic disorder" refers to a more narrow diagnosis defined by criteria in the *Diagnostic and Statistical Manual of Mental Disorders, 4th edition* (DSM-IV-TR) (APA, 2000).

dards, 2000), which can lead to serious illness and death in recipients. In that report, the committee concluded that the evidence was inadequate to accept or reject a causal relationship between exposure to thimerosal from vaccines and the NDDs of autism, attention deficit hyperactivity disorder (ADHD), and speech or language delay. The committee's causality conclusion was based on the fact that there were no published epidemiological studies examining the potential association between TCVs and NDDs, and the two unpublished, epidemiological studies that were available (Blaxill, 2001; Verstraeten, 2001) provided only weak and inconclusive evidence of an association between TCVs and NDDs. The committee also concluded that the hypothesis linking TCVs with NDDs was not yet established and rested on incomplete evidence. However, because mercury is a known neurotoxin, and prenatal exposures to methylmercury (a compound closely related to the form of mercury in TCVs) have been documented to negatively affect early childhood development (see NRC, 2000),[2] a potential biological mechanism could be hypothesized based on analogies with this compound.

New epidemiological studies and biological mechanism theories on both issues have emerged since the publication of these IOM reports. In this report, the committee incorporates the new epidemiological evidence and studies of biologic mechanisms relating to vaccines and autism; it does not address the hypothesized link between vaccines and other NDDs.

Until 1999, thimerosal was contained in over 30 vaccines licensed and marketed in the United States, including some of the vaccines administered to infants for protection against diphtheria, tetanus, pertussis, *Haemophilus influenzae* type b (Hib), and hepatitis B. The controversy over thimerosal in vaccines erupted that year, when FDA researchers determined that under the recommended childhood immunization schedule, infants might be exposed to cumulative doses of ethylmercury that exceed some federal safety guidelines established for ingestion of methylmercury, another form of organic mercury (Ball et al., 2001). In July 1999, the American Academy of Pediatrics (AAP) and the U.S. Public Health Service (PHS) issued a joint statement recommending the removal of thimerosal from vaccines as soon as possible (CDC, 1999). With the licensure of a thimerosal-free hepatitis B vaccine in August 1999 and approval of a thimerosal-free preservative hepatitis B vaccine in March 2000, children had access to a hepatitis B vaccine that did not contain thimerosal as a preservative by March 2000. With the FDA approval of a second thimerosal-free version of DTaP vaccine in March 2001, all formulations of vaccines on the U.S. recommended childhood immunization schedule for children 6 years of age or younger became available free of thimerosal used as a preservative (FDA, 2002). Based on information from vaccine

---

[2]For example, there is evidence that fetal exposure to mercury might lead to detectable differences in neurodevelopmental testing that might be consistent with some neurodevelopmental disabilities (see NRC, 2000).

manufacturers provided to the FDA, the lots of vaccine manufactured before this time that contained thimerosal as a preservative and had been released to the market had expiration dates in 2002 (FDA, 2004). Based on these changes, the maximum amount of mercury from vaccines on the recommended childhood immunization schedule that an infant (less than 6 months of age) can now be exposed to is <3 µg,[3] down from 187.5 µg in 1999 (FDA, 2001, 2004).

The controversy regarding the hypothesized link between the MMR vaccine and autism began in 1998 when Dr. Andrew Wakefield and colleagues published a case series describing 12 children with pervasive developmental disorder associated with gastrointestinal (GI) symptoms and developmental regression (Wakefield et al., 1998). For eight of these children, the onset of their behavioral problems was associated, through retrospective accounts by their parents or physicians, with MMR vaccination. This study put forth a hypothesis that a new phenotype of autism characterized by GI symptoms and developmental regression could be associated with the MMR vaccine. While the authors acknowledged that the study did not prove an association between MMR and the conditions seen in these children, the report generated considerable interest and concern about a possible link between MMR vaccination and ASD—regressive autism in particular. A recent statement from 10 of the original 13 authors states that the data were insufficient to establish a causal link between MMR vaccine and autism (Murch et al., 2004).

Causality Argument

Epidemiological studies examining TCVs and autism, including three controlled observational studies (Hviid et al., 2003; Miller, 2004; Verstraeten et al., 2003) and two uncontrolled observational studies (Madsen et al., 2003; Stehr-Green et al., 2003), consistently provided evidence of no association between TCVs and autism, despite the fact that these studies utilized different methods and examined different populations (in Sweden, Denmark, the United States, and the United Kingdom). Other studies reported findings of an association. These include two ecological studies[4] (Geier and Geier, 2003a, 2004a), three studies using passive reporting data (Geier and Geier, 2003a,b,d) one unpublished study using Vaccine Safety Datalink (VSD) data (Geier and Geier, 2004b,c), and one

---

[3]3µg is the maximum amount that could have been received by an infant in the first 6 months of life if they received trace-containing formulations (e.g., Engerix B hepatitis B vaccine, Tripedia DTaP vaccine) as opposed to those that contain no thimerosal (e.g., Recombivax HB hepatitis B vaccine pediatric formulation, Infanrix DTaP, Daptacel DTaP) (FDA, 2004d).

[4]These studies were classified as ecological because they rely on aggregate data rather than individual-level data to make inferences about causality. However, the authors appear to attempt an individual-level analysis, but it is unclear how this can be, given the data they used. Based on the available information, the study design is indeterminate. See text for more information.

unpublished uncontrolled study (Blaxill, 2001). However, the studies by Geier and Geier cited above have serious methodological flaws and their analytic methods were nontransparent, making their results uninterpretable, and therefore noncontributory with respect to causality (see text for full discussion). The study by Blaxill is uninformative with respect to causality because of its methodological limitations. Thus, based on this body of evidence, **the committee concludes that the evidence favors rejection of a causal relationship between thimerosal-containing vaccines and autism.** This conclusion differs from the committee's finding in its 2001 report on TCVs and NDDs which was that the evidence was "inadequate to accept or reject a causal relationship between exposure to thimerosal from childhood vaccines and the neurodevelopmental disorders of autism, ADHD, and speech and language delay." (IOM, 2001b, p. 66) The committee's conclusion in 2001 was based on the fact that there were no published epidemiological studies examining the potential association between TCVs and NDDs, and the two unpublished, epidemiological studies that were available (Blaxill, 2001; Verstraeten, 2001) provided only weak and inconclusive evidence of an association between TCVs and NDDs. Furthermore, the conclusion in the 2001 report pertained to a broader set of NDDs, while this report's conclusion applies *only* to autism.

Studies examining the association between MMR and autism, including nine controlled observational studies (DeStefano et al., 2004; DeWilde et al., 2001; Farrington et al., 2001; Fombonne and Chakrabarti, 2001; Madsen et al., 2002; Makela et al., 2002; Takahashi et al., 2003; Taylor et al., 1999, 2002), three ecological studies (Dales et al., 2001; Gillberg and Heijbel, 1998; Kaye et al., 2001), and two studies based on passive reporting system in Finland (Patja et al., 2000; Peltola et al., 1998), consistently showed evidence of no association between the MMR vaccine and autism. Two studies reported findings of a positive association between MMR and autism. The first was an ecological study (Geier and Geier, 2004a) that reported a potential positive correlation between the number of doses of measles-containing vaccine and the cases of autism reported to the special education system in the 1980s. The second was a study of passive reporting data by the same authors (Geier and Geier, 2003c) that reported a positive correlation between autism reports in the Vaccine Adverse Events Reporting System (VAERS) and estimated administered doses of MMR. However, these two studies are characterized by serious methodological flaws and their analytic methods were nontransparent, making their results uninterpretable, and therefore noncontributory with respect to causality (see text for full discussion). The case series study by Wakefield and colleagues (Wakefield et al., 1998), which originally raised the hypothesis linking MMR and autism, is uninformative with respect to causality. Based on this body of evidence, **the committee concludes that the evidence favors rejection of a causal relationship between MMR vaccine and autism.** This conclusion is consistent with the finding in the committee's previous report on MMR and autism (IOM, 2001a).

Biological Mechanisms

Autism is a very complex disorder. A strong genetic component clearly exists, but there is a growing understanding that environmental factors might be important contributors to the expression of that genetic susceptibility. Animal models (primarily rat models), clinical observations, and pathological data point to an array of possible pathways by which autism develops, though none are proven. Many different pathways might lead to similar expressions, which could account for the multiple presentations of autism.

A link between vaccine components, such as the measles vaccine-strain virus or the ethylmercury preservative thimerosal, is difficult to establish because of the early stage of scientific understanding about the cause(s) of autism. The committee read, and heard presentations at their workshop, about several hypotheses. Data presented to support these hypotheses derive from rodent models of human autism, observations of abnormalities in children with autism or their families, and *in vitro* studies.

One hypothesis about the MMR vaccine involves the presence of measles virus lodging in the intestine of some children, which releases gut-brain mediators or toxins, leading to autism (Wakefield et al., 2002). Another hypothesis related to MMR vaccine is that children with autism have immune abnormalities that are indicative of vaccine-induced-central-nervous system, immune-mediated damage that leads to autism (Singh, 2004).

The thimerosal-related hypothesis is that some genetically susceptible population of children react to the thimerosal in vaccines with increased accumulation and decreased excretion of mercury from the brain, which alters several key biochemical pathways—for example, apoptosis and DNA metabolism—leading to autism (Bradstreet, 2004). A genetically susceptible subset of children who develop autism following vaccinations is offered as one theoretical explanation for the findings in epidemiological studies of no association between vaccination and autism.

Autism is a heterogeneous syndrome with a broad range of behavioral symptoms and severity. As yet, a biological marker specific for autism has not been defined. It is thus possible that autism encompasses a spectrum of disease subtypes that have different etiologies. This may explain the wide range of immunological abnormalities that have been found in the serum of patients with autism, with some studies reporting evidence of decreased cell-mediated immunity (CMI), and others reporting increased/overactive CMI. Other support for an association of autism with immune dysfunction includes the increased frequency of an extended major histocompatibility complex (MHC) haplotype in autism, increased autoantibodies to brain antigens, and the increased incidence of autoimmune diseases noted in a retrospective study of relatives of people with autism.

However, despite evidence of immune dysregulation in the serum of people with autism, there is as yet no evidence that the immune system plays a direct role in the neuropathogenesis of autism. Unlike neuroimmunological diseases such as multiple sclerosis, there is no evidence of immune activation or inflammatory lesions in the brains or cerebrospinal fluid of people with autism. This fact also makes it likely that a link with MMR vaccination is circumstantial rather than causal.

It is clear from twin and family studies that there is a strong genetic basis for autism. The recent discovery of the genetic basis of Rett's syndrome, a phenotypically similar NDD with similarly described immunological abnormalities, may shed some light on the pathogenesis of autism. Similar epigenetic mechanisms may be operating in autism that lead to simultaneously abnormal development in the immune and central nervous systems.

The hypothesis reviewed by the committee is that vaccine-induced autism represents the end result of a combination of susceptibility (possibly genetic) to immune dysfunction or to abnormal mercury metabolism. Posited intermediate steps include enzymatic abnormalities that might be related to the apoptosis and cellular signaling, leading to an array of behavioral, cognitive, sensory, and motor disturbances. Other environmental exposures have similar effects.

Rodent models suggest that reactions to some infectious agents (e.g., bornavirus and group A streptococcus) lead to somewhat specific neuronal cell death and evidence of autoimmune reactions in the developing and adult brains of rodents. The animals also exhibit abnormal behaviors. These immunological and behavioral findings are similar to those seen in some humans after infection: the behavior in children with PANDAS or in the animal models resembles the behavior constellations in children with autism. A similar set of comparisons can be made with mercury exposures (Bernard et al., 2001), although autism has never been documented as a consequence of high-dose mercury exposure, including acrodynia. While analogies are useful for hypothesis generation, they do not substitute for direct evidence.

Other evidence offered for the vaccine-autism hypothesis includes analogies between rodent behavior and human behavior as well as clinical observations of metabolic or immunologic differences between individuals with autism and normal subjects or subjects with other conditions. In the clinical studies, it is not clear to what extent the abnormalities are antecedents or are comorbid disease expressions, rather than causal factors. That is, it is possible that some people with autism, perhaps even a subgroup that could be identified at some time in the future by genetic markers, also have abnormal immune reactions and abnormal mercury metabolism but that vaccination does not cause these abnormalities, nor do they cause autism.

The committee notes several factors that limit acceptance at this time of the hypothesis that vaccines cause autism. The evidence offered for the hypothesis includes data from *in vitro* experimental systems, analogies between rodent behavior, and human behavior and clinical observations that are at least as well explained as being comorbid disease expressions than as causal factors. That is, it is possible that some people with autism, perhaps even a subgroup that could eventually be identified by genetic markers, have abnormal immune reactions and abnormal mercury metabolism, but that vaccination of these individuals does not cause these abnormalities or autism itself. However, the experiments showing effects of thimerosal on biochemical pathways in cell culture systems and showing abnormalities in the immune system or metal metabolism in people with autism are provocative; the autism research community should consider the appropriate composition of the autism research portfolio with some of these new findings in mind. However, these experiments do not provide evidence of a relationship between vaccines or thimerosal and autism.

In the absence of experimental or human evidence that vaccination (either the MMR vaccine or the preservative thimerosal) affects metabolic, developmental, immune, or other physiological or molecular mechanisms that are causally related to the development of autism, the committee concludes that the hypotheses generated to date are theoretical only.

SIGNIFICANCE ASSESSMENT

Autism leads to substantial challenges for the families of affected individuals because many people with autism remain dependent throughout their lives. Special education costs can exceed $30,000 per year. The annual cost of care in a residential school may be as much as $80,000-100,000 (CDC, 1999). In addition to the substantial financial strains, families of children with autism face other demands. During the committees' public session in March 2001 and in the material submitted for the February 2004 meeting, the committee heard about the difficulties of caring for children with autism. Parents described round-the-clock efforts to care for their child, the difficulty of finding knowledgeable and sympathetic health care providers, the challenges in finding high-quality information, and the frustrations of seeing their child change from being active and engaged to being aloof and nonresponsive. Many clinicians, including several committee members, have treated children with autism and witnessed the difficulties and pain experienced by the children and their families.

Although autism is recognized as a serious condition and strides have been made in understanding the disease in many areas, significant gaps remain, particularly regarding its etiology and risk factors. These gaps include uncertainty about prevalence and incidence trends; limited knowledge of the natural history of autism, including its early onset and regressive forms; the lack of a strong biological model for autism; limited understanding of potentially associated features (e.g., immune alterations, enterocolitis); and no current basis for identifying possible subtypes of autism with different pathogeneses related to genetic and environmental interactions. Research has been hindered by changing case definitions and the heterogeneity of study populations that may include cases linked to other known medical risk factors (e.g., Fragile X).

The hypothesis that vaccines, specifically MMR vaccine and the preservative thimerosal, cause autism is among the most contentious of issues reviewed by vaccine safety committees of the IOM. One needs to read just one of the many websites and Internet-based discussion groups on the issue of autism[5] to get a picture of the complicated lives of families with children with autism and the anger of some families toward the federal government (particularly the CDC and FDA), vaccine manufacturers, the field of epidemiology, and traditional biomedical research. The volume of correspondence to the committee on this issue is impassioned and impressive. There are, however, little data to shed light on how many families believe that vaccination actually caused their child's autism,[6] so that the magnitude of concern in the general population is uncertain. **However, the committee concludes that because autism can be such a devastating disease, any speculation that links vaccines and autism means that this is a significant issue.**

There are many examples in medicine of disorders defined by a constellation of symptoms that have multiple etiologies, and autism is likely to be among them. Determining a specific cause in the individual is impossible unless the etiology is known and there is a biological marker. Determining causality with population-based methods such as epidemiological analyses requires either a well-defined at-risk population or a large effect in the general population. Absent biomarkers, well-defined risk factors, or large effect sizes, the committee cannot rule out, based on the epidemiological evidence, the possibility that vaccines contribute to autism in some small subset or very unusual circumstances. However, there is currently no evidence to support this hypothesis either.

The committee concludes that much more research must be conducted on autism. However, research should be directed towards those lines of inquiry most supported by the current state of knowledge. The vaccine hypotheses are not currently supported by the evidence. Much remains unknown about the etiology or etiologies of autism. Furthermore, there have not been many studies on treatments for autism. Research should be directed towards better understanding the etiology or etiologies of autism and on treatments for autism.

While the committee strongly supports targeted research that focuses on better understanding the disease of autism, from a public health perspective the committee does not consider a significant investment in studies of the theoretical vaccine-autism connection to be useful at this time. The nature of the debate about vaccine safety now includes the theory by some that genetic susceptibility makes vaccinations risky for some people, which calls into question the appropriateness of a public health, or universal, vaccination strategy. However, the benefits of vaccination are proven and the hypothesis of susceptible populations is

---

[5]See http://health.groups.yahoo.com/group/Autism-Mercury/messages.

[6]Over three thousand families have filed claims for compensation for autism with the Vaccine Injury Compensation Program (VICP).

presently speculative. Using an unsubstantiated hypothesis to question the safety of vaccination and the ethical behavior of those governmental agencies and scientists who advocate for vaccination could lead to widespread rejection of vaccines and inevitable increases in incidences of serious infectious diseases like measles, whooping cough, and Hib bacterial meningitis.

The committee encourages that research on autism focus more broadly on the disorders' causes of and treatments for it. Thus, **the committee recommends a public health response that fully supports an array of vaccine safety activities. In addition the committee recommends that available funding for autism research be channeled to the most promising areas.**

The committee emphasizes that confidence in the safety of vaccines is essential to an effective immunization program—one that provides maximum protection against vaccine-preventable diseases with the safest vaccines possible. Questions about vaccine safety must be addressed responsibly by public health officials, health professionals, and vaccine manufacturers. Although the hypotheses related to vaccines and autism will remain highly salient to some individuals, (parents, physicians, and researchers), this concern must be balanced against the broader benefit of the current vaccine program for all children.

RECOMMENDATIONS FOR PUBLIC HEALTH RESPONSE

Specific recommendations regarding policy review, epidemiologic research and surveillance, and communication follow. The committee also revisits and discusses many of the recommendations of its two previous reports on vaccines and autism (IOM, 2001a,b).

Policy Review

- **At this time, the committee does not recommend a policy review of the licensure of MMR vaccine or of the current schedule and recommendations for the administration of the MMR vaccine.**
- **At this time, the committee does not recommend a policy review of the current schedule and recommendations for the administration of routine childhood vaccines based on hypotheses regarding thimerosal and autism.** Currently, thimerosal has been removed from all universally recommended childhood vaccines except influenza vaccine. A thimerosal-free version of the influenza vaccine exists, however, and is available for use in infants, children, and pregnant women. There are a few vaccines with thimerosal (e.g., Td) that infants and young children[7] could be exposed to, but only under very special circumstances.

---

[7]Td is recommended for children 12-18, but it is conceivable that some infants and young children could receive Td in lieu of DTaP.

• The committee also recommended in its prior report that the appropriate professional societies and government agencies review their policies on the non-vaccine biological and pharmaceutical products that contain thimerosal and are used in infants, children, and pregnant women. The committee's recommendation reflected concern about total mercury burden and potential risk of certain NDDs. While the United States chose to eliminate thimerosal from routine childhood vaccines as a precautionary measure and because it was feasible, the committee recognizes that other countries have different constraints and other factors; their own assessments of the risks and benefits may lead those countries to reach different conclusions regarding the thimerosal content of their vaccines. **Given the lack of direct evidence for a biological mechanism and the fact that all well-designed epidemiological studies provide evidence of no association between thimerosal and autism, the committee recommends that cost-benefit assessments regarding the use of thimerosal-containing versus thimerosal-free vaccines and other biological or pharmaceutical products, whether in the United States or other countries, should not include autism as a potential risk.**

Surveillance and Epidemiologic Research

• **The committee reaffirms its previous recommendation to use standard and accepted case definitions and assessment protocols for ASD to enhance the precision and comparability of results from surveillance, epidemiological studies, and biological investigations. Studies should also address the heterogeneity in the etiology of ASD and the spectrum of clinical presentation.**

• **The committee reaffirms its previous recommendation to conduct clinical and epidemiological studies of sufficient rigor to identify risk factors and biological markers of ASD in order to better understand genetic or environmental causes of ASD.**

• **Surveillance of adverse events related to vaccines is important and should be strengthened in several ways:**

  — **The committee recommends that standardized case definitions for adverse events be adopted.**

  — **The committee recommends that formal guidelines or criteria be developed for using VAERS data to study adverse events.**

  — **The committee recommends the continued use of large-linked databases, active surveillance, and other tools to evaluate potential vaccine-related adverse events.**

  — **The committee supports the development of Clinical Immunization Safety Assessment (CISA) centers to improve understanding of adverse events at the individual level.**

- Many of the epidemiological research recommendations of the committee's 2001 report on thimerosal and NDDs are either under way or have been completed. **Insofar as monitoring of ASD occurs, one area of complementary research that the committee continues to recommend is surveillance of ASD as exposure to thimerosal declines.** Any research in this area should be conducted with critical attention to case definition, diagnostic criteria, and other factors (for example, data collection procedures and definitions of autism in the special education system) that could affect prevalence estimates of ASD.

- Little is known about the levels of background exposure to mercury in the population. **The committee recommends increased efforts to quantify the level of prenatal and postnatal exposure to thimerosal and other forms of mercury in infants, children, and pregnant women.**

Clinical Studies

- The committee heard from some parents of children with ASD who have chosen to rely on chelation therapy as a treatment. The committee saw no scientific evidence, however, that chelation is an effective therapy for ASD or is even indicated in these circumstances. Chelation therapy is currently indicated only for high-dose, acute mercury poisonings. **Because chelation therapy has potentially serious risks, the committee recommends that it be used only in carefully controlled research settings with appropriate oversight by Institutional Review Boards protecting the interests of the children who participate.**

Communication

Many parents described to the committee their concerns about the MMR vaccine and thimerosal use in vaccines. Many expressed their frustration and difficulties in making informed decisions about vaccination of their children as their level of trust in the government, media, and science in general has declined. Because of the importance and difficulty of maintaining mutual trust, a model that focuses on increasing public participation in risk decisionmaking is likely to make that process more democratic and improve the relevance and quality of the technical analysis (Slovic, 1999). Such participative processes may not necessarily lead to increased acceptability of risk policies, but may lead to higher quality decision-making processes (Arvai, 2003). However, better risk-benefit communication requires attention to the needs of both the scientific and public communities. Many scientists need to develop a more comprehensive understanding of what risk-benefit communication entails and the rich knowledge base that can be used to design strategic communication programs. Appreciating that risk-benefit communication requires two-way exchanges of information and opinions (NRC,

1989) and working from a larger frame of communication methods, scientists will be able to work more effectively with the public to address vaccine-related issues. A mix of information, dissemination, education services, and community-based dialogues are probably needed (NRC, 1989).

To address these goals, **the committee recommends developing programs to increase public participation in vaccine safety research and policy decisions and to enhance the skills and willingness of scientists and government officials to engage in constructive dialogue with the public about research findings and their implications for policy development.** Programs such as Project LEAD®, COPUS Grant Schemes, or the IOM Vaccine Safety Forum may serve as useful models. Any proposed program should be easily accessible to the public and should involve a wide range of individuals. Additionally, ways to rebuild trust between the public, scientists, professionals, media, and government should be explored.

BOX ES-1
Committee Conclusions and Recommendations

SCIENTIFIC ASSESSMENT
Causality Conclusions

The committee concludes that the evidence favors rejection of a causal relationship between thimerosal-containing vaccines and autism.

The committee concludes that the evidence favors rejection of a causal relationship between MMR vaccine and autism.

Biological Mechanisms Conclusions

In the absence of experimental or human evidence that vaccination (either the MMR vaccine or the preservative thimerosal) affects metabolic, developmental, immune, or other physiological or molecular mechanisms that are causally related to the development of autism, the committee concludes that the hypotheses generated to date are theoretical only.

SIGNIFICANCE ASSESSMENT

The committee concludes that because autism can be such a devastating disease, any speculation that links vaccines and autism means that this is a significant issue.

PUBLIC HEALTH RESPONSE RECOMMENDATIONS

The committee recommends a public health response that fully supports an array of vaccine safety activities. In addition the committee recommends that available funding for autism research be channeled to the most promising areas.

Policy Review

At this time, the committee does not recommend a policy review of the licensure of MMR vaccine or of the current schedule and recommendations for the administration of the MMR vaccine.

At this time, the committee does not recommend a policy review of the current schedule and recommendations for the administration of routine childhood vaccines based on hypotheses regarding thimerosal and autism.

Given the lack of direct evidence for a biological mechanism and the fact that all well-designed epidemiological studies provide evidence of no association between thimerosal and autism, the committee recommends that cost-benefit assessments regarding the use of thimerosal-containing versus thimerosal-free vaccines and other biological or pharmaceutical products, whether in the United States or other countries, should not include autism as a potential risk.

Surveillance and Epidemiologic Research

The committee reaffirms its previous recommendation to use standard and accepted case definitions and assessment protocols for ASD to enhance the precision and comparability of results from surveillance, epidemiological studies, and biological investigations. Studies should also address the heterogeneity in the etiology of ASD and the spectrum of clinical presentation.

The committee reaffirms its previous recommendation to conduct clinical and epidemiological studies of sufficient rigor to identify risk factors and biological markers of ASD in order to better understand genetic or environmental causes of ASD.

Surveillance of adverse events related to vaccines is important and should be strengthened in several ways:

The committee recommends that standardized case definitions for adverse events be adopted.

The committee recommends that formal guidelines or criteria be developed for using VAERS data to study adverse events.

The committee recommends the continued use of large-linked databases, active surveillance, and other tools to evaluate potential vaccine-related adverse events.

The committee supports the development of Clinical Immunization Safety Assessment (CISA) centers to improve understanding of adverse events at the individual level.

One area of complementary research that the committee continues to recommend is surveillance of ASD as exposure to thimerosal declines.

The committee recommends increased efforts to quantify the level of prenatal and postnatal exposure to thimerosal and other forms of mercury in infants, children, and pregnant women.

Clinical Studies

Because chelation therapy has potentially serious risks, the committee recommends that it be used only in carefully-controlled research settings with appropriate oversight by Institutional Review Boards protecting the interests of the children who participate.

Communication

Better risk-benefit communication requires attention to the needs of both the scientific community and public communities. Many scientists need to develop a more comprehensive understanding of what risk-benefit communication entails and the rich knowledge base that can be used to design strategic communication programs. Thus, the committee recommends developing programs to increase public participation in vaccine safety research and policy decisions and to enhance the skills and willingness of scientists and government officials to engage in constructive dialogue with the public about research findings and their implications for policy development.

REFERENCES

APA (American Psychiatric Association). 1994. *Diagnostic and Statistical Manual of Mental Disorders*. 4th ed. Washington, DC: APA.

APA. 2000. *Diagnostic and Statistical Manual of Mental Disorders; Text Revision*. 4th ed. Washington, DC: APA.

Arvai JL. 2003. Using risk communication to disclose the outcome of a participatory decision-making process: effects on the perceived acceptability of risk-policy decisions. *Risk Anal* 23(2):281-9.

Ball LK, Ball R, Pratt RD. 2001. An assessment of thimerosal use in childhood vaccines. *Pediatrics* 107(5):1147-54.

Bernard S, Enayati A, Redwood L, Roger H, Binstock T. 2001. Autism: a novel form of mercury poisoning. *Med Hypotheses* 56(4):462-71.

Blaxill M. 2001. Presentation to the Immunization Safety Review Committee. *Rising Incidence of Autism: Association with Thimerosal*. Cambridge, MA.

Bradstreet J. 2004. Presentation to the Immunization Safety Review Committee. *Biological Evidence of Significant Vaccine Related Side-effects Resulting in Neurodevelopmental Disorders*. Washington, DC.

CDC (Centers for Disease Control and Prevention). 1999. Thimerosal in vaccines: a joint statement of the American Academy of Pediatrics and the Public Health Service. *Morb Mortal Wkly Rep* 48(26):563-5.

Dales L, Hammer SJ, Smith N. 2001. Time trends in autism and in MMR immunization coverage in California. *JAMA* 285(9):1183-5.

DeStefano F, Bhasin TK, Thompson WW, Yeargin-Allsopp M, Boyle C. 2004. Age at first measles-mumps-rubella vaccination in children with autism and school-matched control subjects: a population-based study in metropolitan Atlanta. *Pediatrics* 113(2):259-66.

DeWilde S, Carey IM, Richards N, Hilton SR, Cook DG. 2001. Do children who become autistic consult more often after MMR vaccination? *British J General Practice* 51(464):226-7.

Farrington CP, Miller E, Taylor B. 2001. MMR and autism: further evidence against a causal association. *Vaccine* 19(27):3632-5.

FDA (Food and Drug Administration). 2001. Thimerosal content in some currently manufactured U.S. Licensed vaccines (table). [Online] Available: URL http://www.fda.gov/cber/vaccine/thimcnt.htm [accessed July, 2001].

FDA. 2004. Thimerosal content in vaccines. (Email communication from Karen Midthun, Food and Drug Administration, May 7, 2004).

Filipek PA, Accardo PJ, Baranek GT, Cook EH, Dawson G, Gordon B, Gravel JS, Johnson CP, Kallen RJ, Levy SE, Minshew NJ, Ozonoff S, Prizant BM, Rapin I, Rogers SJ, Stone WL, Teplin S, Tuchman RF, Volkmar FR. 1999. The screening and diagnosis of autistic spectrum disorders. *J Autism Dev Disord* 29(6):439-84.

Fombonne E. 1999. The epidemiology of autism: a review. *Psychol Med* 29(4):769-86.

Fombonne E, Chakrabarti S. 2001. No evidence for a new variant of measles-mumps-rubella-induced autism. *Pediatrics* 108(4):E58.

Fombonne E. 2003. The prevalence of autism. *JAMA* 289(1):87-9.

Geier DA, Geier MR. 2003a. An assessment of the impact of thimerosal on childhood neurodevelopmental disorders. *Pediatr Rehabil* 6(2):97-102.

Geier M, Geier D. 2003b. Neurodevelopmental disorders after thimerosal-containing vaccines: a brief communication. *Exp Biol Med (Maywood)* 228(6):660-4.

Geier M, Geier D. 2003c. Pediatric MMR vaccination safety. *International Pediatrics* 18(2):203-8.

Geier MR, Geier DA. 2003d. Thimerosal in childhood vaccines, neurodevelopmental disorders, and heart disease in the United States. *J Amer Phys Sur* 8(1):6-11.

Geier DA, Geier MR. 2004a. A comparative evaluation of the effects of MMR immunization and mercury doses from thimerosal-containing childhood vaccines on the population prevalence of autism. *Med Sci Monit* 10(3):PI33-9.

Geier D, Geier M. 2004b. *Presentation to the Immunization Safety Review Committee.* From Epidemiology, Clinical Medicine, Molecular Biology, and Atoms, to Politics: A Review of the Relationship between Thimerosal and Autism. Washington, DC.

Geier D, Geier M. 2004c. Submission to the Immunization Safety Review Committee. *From Epidemiology, Clinical Medicine, Molecular Biology, and Atoms, to Politics: A Review of the Relationship Between Thimerosal and Autism.*

General Biologics Product Standards. 2000. Constituent materials. *21 CFR.* 2000;610.15.

Gillberg C, Heijbel H. 1998. MMR and autism. *Autism.* 2:423-4.

Gillberg C, Wing L. 1999. Autism: not an extremely rare disorder. *Acta Psychiatr Scand* 99(6):399-406.

Hill AB. 1965. The environment and disease: association or causation? *Proc R Soc Med* 58:295-300.

Hviid A, Stellfeld M, Wohlfahrt J, Melbye M. 2003. Association between thimerosal-containing vaccine and autism. *JAMA* 290(13):1763-6.

IOM (Institute of Medicine). 1991. *Adverse Events Following Pertussis and Rubella Vaccines.* Washington, DC: National Academy Press.

IOM. 1994. *Adverse Events Associated with Childhood Vaccines: Evidence Bearing on Causality.* Washington, DC: National Academy Press.

IOM. 2001a. *Immunization Safety Review: Measles-Mumps-Rubella Vaccine and Autism.* Washington, DC: National Academy Press.

IOM. 2001b. *Immunization Safety Review: Thimerosal-Containing Vaccines and Neurodevelopmental Disorders.* Washington, DC: National Academy Press.

IOM. 2002. *Immunization Safety Review: Multiple Immunizations and Immune Dysfunction.* Washington, DC: National Academy Press.

Kaye JA, del Mar Melero-Montes M, Jick H. 2001. Mumps, measles, and rubella vaccine and the incidence of autism recorded by general practitioners: a time trend analysis. *British Med J* 322(7284):460-3.

Madsen KM, Hviid A, Vestergaard M, Schendel D, Wohlfahrt J, Thorsen P, Olsen J, Melbye M. 2002. A population-based study of measles, mumps, and rubella vaccination and autism. *N Engl J Med* 347(19):1477-82.

Madsen KM, Lauritsen MB, Pedersen CB, Thorsen P, Plesner AM, Andersen PH, Mortensen PB. 2003. Thimerosal and the occurrence of autism: negative ecological evidence from Danish population-based data. *Pediatrics* 112(3 Pt 1):604-6.

Makela A, Nuorti JP, Peltola H. 2002. Neurologic disorders after measles-mumps-rubella vaccination. *Pediatrics* 110(5):957-63.

Miller E. 2004. Presentation to the Immunization Safety Review Committee. *Thimerosal and Developmental Problems Including Autism.* Washington, DC.

Murch SH, Anthony A, Casson DH, Malik M, Berelowitz M, Dhillon AP, Thomson MA, Valentine A, Davies SE, Walker-Smith JA. 2004. Retraction of an interpretation. *Lancet* 363:750.

NRC (National Research Council). 1989. *Improving Risk Communication.* Washington DC: National Academy Press.

NRC. 2000. *Toxicological Effects of Methylmercury.* Washington, DC: National Academy Press.

Patja A, Davidkin I, Kurki T, Kallio MJ, Valle M, Peltola H. 2000. Serious adverse events after measles-mumps-rubella vaccination during a fourteen-year prospective follow-up. *Pediatr Infect Dis J* 19(12):1127-34.

Peltola H, Patja A, Leinikki P, Valle M, Davidkin I, Paunio M. 1998. No evidence for measles, mumps, and rubella vaccine-associated inflammatory bowel disease or autism in a 14-year prospective study [letter]. *Lancet* 351(9112):1327-8.

Singh VK. 2004. Submission to the Immunization Safety Review. *Autism, Vaccines, and Immune Reactions*. Utah State University: Logan, UT.

Slovic P. 1999. Trust, emotion, sex, politics, and science: surveying the risk-assessment battlefield. *Risk Anal* 19(4):689-701.

Stehr-Green P, Tull P, Stellfeld M, Mortenson PB, Simpson D. 2003. Autism and thimerosal-containing vaccines: lack of consistent evidence for an association. *Am J Prev Med* 25(2):101-6.

Takahashi H, Suzumura S, Shirakizawa F, Wada N, Tanaka-Taya K, Arai S, Okabe N, Ichikawa H, Sato T. 2003. An epidemiological study on Japanese autism concerning routine childhood immunization history. *Jpn J Infect Dis* 56(3):114-7.

Taylor B, Miller E, Farrington CP, Petropoulos MC, Favot-Mayaud I, Li J, Waight PA. 1999. Autism and measles, mumps, and rubella vaccine: no epidemiological evidence for a causal association. *Lancet* 353(9169):2026-9.

Taylor B, Miller E, Lingam R, Andrews N, Simmons ASJ. 2002. Measles, mumps, and rubella vaccination and bowel problems or developmental regression in children with autism: population study. *British Med J* 324(7334):393-6.

Verstraeten T. 2001. Presentation to Immunization Safety Review Committee. *Vaccine Safety Datalink (VSD) Screening Study and Follow-Up Analysis with Harvard Pilgrim Data.* Cambridge, Massachusetts.

Verstraeten T, Davis RL, DeStefano F, Lieu TA, Rhodes PH, Black SB, Shinefield H, Chen RT, Vaccine Safety Datalink Team. 2003. Safety of thimerosal-containing vaccines: a two-phased study of computerized health maintenance organization databases. *Pediatrics* 112(5):1039-48.

Volkmar F, Pauls D. 2003. Autism. *Lancet* 362:1133-1141.

Wakefield AJ, Murch SH, Anthony A, Linnell J, Casson DM, Malik M, Berelowitz M, Dhillon AP, Thomson MA, Harvey P, Valentine A, Davies SE, Walker-Smith JA. 1998. Ileal-lymphoid-nodular hyperplasia, non-specific colitis, and pervasive developmental disorder in children. *Lancet* 351(9103):637-41.

Wakefield AJ, Puleston JM, Montgomery SM, Anthony A, O'Leary JJ, Murch SH. 2002. Review article: the concept of entero-colonic encephalopathy, autism and opioid receptor ligands. *Aliment Pharmacol Ther* 16(4):663-74.

Immunization Safety Review: Vaccines and Autism

Immunization to protect children and adults from infectious diseases is one of the greatest achievements of public health. Immunization is not without risks, however. It is well established, for example, that the oral polio vaccine on rare occasion has caused paralytic polio and that vaccines sometimes produce anaphylactic shock. Given the widespread use of vaccines, state mandates requiring vaccination of children for entry into school, college, or day care, and the importance of ensuring that trust in immunization programs is justified, it is essential that safety concerns receive assiduous attention.

The Immunization Safety Review Committee was established by the Institute of Medicine (IOM) to evaluate the evidence on possible causal associations between immunizations and certain adverse outcomes, and to then present conclusions and recommendations. The committee's mandate also includes assessing the broader significance for society of these immunization safety issues.

This eighth report from the committee examines the hypothesis that vaccines, specifically the measles-mumps-rubella (MMR) vaccine and thimerosal-containing vaccines, are associated with autism.

THE CHARGE TO THE COMMITTEE

Challenges to the safety of immunizations are prominent in public and scientific debate. Given these persistent and growing concerns, the Centers for Disease Control and Prevention (CDC) and the National Institutes of Health (NIH) recognized the need for an independent, expert group to address immunization safety in a timely and objective manner. The IOM has been involved in such issues since the 1970s. (A brief chronology can be found in Appendix D.) In 1999, because of IOM's previous work and its access to independent scientific experts, CDC and NIH began a year of discussions with IOM to develop the Immunization Safety Review project, which would address both existing and emerging vaccine safety issues.

The Immunization Safety Review Committee is responsible for examining a broad variety of immunization safety concerns. Committee members have expertise in pediatrics, neurology, immunology, internal medicine, infectious diseases, genetics, epidemiology, biostatistics, risk perception and communication, decision analysis, public health, nursing, and ethics. While all of the committee members share the view that immunization is generally beneficial, none of them has a vested interest in the specific immunization safety issues that come before the group. Additional discussion of the committee composition can be found in the Foreword, written by Dr. Harvey Fineberg, President of the IOM.

The committee was charged with examining up to three immunization safety hypotheses each year during the three-year study period (2001-2003). These hypotheses were selected by the Interagency Vaccine Group (IAVG), whose members represent several units of the Department of Health and Human Services: the CDC's National Vaccine Program Office, National Immunization Program, and National Center for Infectious Diseases; the NIH's National Institute of Allergy and Infectious Diseases; the Food and Drug Administration (FDA); the Health Resources and Services Administration's National Vaccine Injury Compensation Program; and the Centers for Medicare & Medicaid Services. The IAVG includes representation from the Department of Defense and the Agency for International Development as well. The committee has issued seven previous reports on vaccine safety issues over the three-year study period (2001-2003). This eighth and final report from the committee examines the hypothesis that vaccines, specifically the MMR vaccine and thimerosal-containing vaccines (TCVs), cause autism. In its first two reports that were published in 2001, the committee examined the hypothesized causal association between the MMR vaccine and autism and TCVs and neurodevelopmental disorders (NDDs), respectively. The IAVG asked the committee to revisit the hypothesized causal association between vaccines and autism in its final report in order to update its conclusions and recommendations based on the significant number of studies that have been undertaken in the last three years.

For each topic, the Immunization Safety Review Committee reviews relevant literature and submissions by interested parties, holds an open scientific meeting, and directly follows the open meeting with a one- to two-day closed meeting to formulate its conclusions and recommendations. The committee's findings are released to the public in a brief consensus report 60 to 90 days after its meeting.

The committee is charged with assessing both the scientific evidence regarding the hypotheses under review and the significance of the issues for society.

- The *scientific* assessment has two components: (1) an examination of the epidemiologic and clinical evidence regarding a possible *causal relationship* between exposure to the vaccine and the adverse event; and (2) an examination of theory, and of experimental or observational evidence from *in vitro*, animal, or human studies, regarding *biological mechanisms* that might be relevant to the hypothesis.
- The *significance* assessment addresses such considerations as the burden of the health risks associated with the adverse event as well as with the vaccine-preventable disease. Other considerations may include the perceived intensity of public or professional concern, and the feasibility of additional research to help resolve scientific uncertainty regarding causality.

The findings of the scientific and significance assessments underlie the committee's recommendations regarding the public health response to the issue. In particular, the committee addresses any needs for a review of immunization policy, for current and future research, and for effective communication strategies. See Figure 1 for a schematic representation of the committee's charge.

THE STUDY PROCESS

The committee held an initial organizational meeting in January 2001. CDC and NIH presented the committee's charge at the meeting, and the committee then conducted a general review of immunization safety concerns. At this meeting, the committee also determined the basic methodology to be used for assessing causality in the hypotheses to be considered in its subsequent deliberations. A website (www.iom.edu/imsafety) and a listserv were created to provide public access to information about the committee's work and to facilitate communication with the committee. The conclusions and recommendations of the committee's reports thus far (see Box 1) are summarized in Appendix A.

For its evaluation of the questions concerning vaccines and autism, the committee held an open scientific meeting in February 2004 to hear presentations on issues germane to the topic (see Appendix B). Many of these presentations are available in electronic form (audio files and slides) on the project website. In addition, the committee reviewed an extensive collection of material, primarily from the published, peer-reviewed scientific and medical literature. The committee also commissioned a paper on autism and the immune system. A list of the

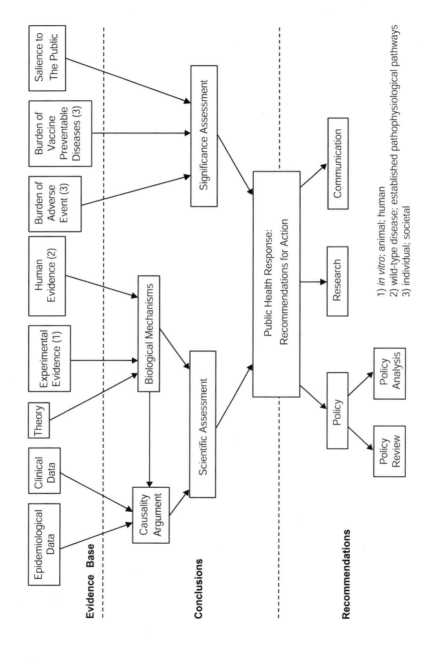

FIGURE 1 Committee charge.

BOX 1
Previous Reports of the
Immunization Safety Review Committee

Immunization Safety Review: Measles-Mumps-Rubella Vaccine and Autism (IOM, 2001a)

Immunization Safety Review: Thimerosal-Containing Vaccines and Neurodevelopmental Disorders (IOM, 2001b)

Immunization Safety Review: Multiple Immunizations and Immune Dysfunction (IOM, 2002b)

Immunization Safety Review: Hepatitis B Vaccine and Demyelinating Neurological Disorders (IOM, 2002a)

Immunization Safety Review: SV40 Contamination of Polio Vaccine and Cancer (IOM, 2002c)

Immunization Safety Review: Vaccinations and Sudden Unexpected Death in Infancy (IOM, 2003)

Immunization Safety Review: Influenza Vaccines and Neurological Complications (IOM, 2004)

---

materials reviewed by the committee, including many items not cited in this report, can be found on the project's website.

THE FRAMEWORK FOR SCIENTIFIC ASSESSMENT

Causality

The Immunization Safety Review Committee has adopted the framework for assessing causality developed by previous IOM committees (IOM, 1991, 1994a,b) convened under the congressional mandate of P.L. 99-660 to address questions of immunization safety. The categories of causal conclusions used by the committee are as follows:

1. No evidence
2. Evidence is inadequate to accept or reject a causal relationship
3. Evidence favors rejection of a causal relationship
4. Evidence favors acceptance of a causal relationship
5. Evidence establishes a causal relationship

Assessments begin from a position of neutrality regarding the specific immunization safety hypothesis under review. That is, there is no presumption that a specific vaccine (or vaccine component) does or does not cause the adverse event in question. The weight of the available clinical and epidemiologic evidence determines whether it is possible to shift from that neutral position to a finding for causality ("the evidence favors acceptance of a causal relationship") or against causality ("the evidence favors rejection of a causal relationship"). The committee does not conclude that the vaccine does not cause the adverse event *merely* because the evidence is inadequate to support causality. Instead, it maintains a neutral position, concluding that the "evidence is inadequate to accept or reject a causal relationship."

Although no firm rules establish the amount of evidence or the quality of the evidence required to support a specific category of causality conclusion, the committee uses standard epidemiologic criteria to guide its decisions. The most definitive category is "establishes causality," which is reserved for those relationships in which the causal link is unequivocal, as with the oral polio vaccine and vaccine-associated paralytic polio or with anaphylactic reactions to vaccine administration (IOM 1991, 1994a). The next category, "favors acceptance" of a causal relationship, reflects evidence that is strong and generally convincing, although not firm enough to be described as unequivocal or established. "Favors rejection" is the strongest category in the negative direction. (The category of "establishes no causal relationship" is *not* used because it is virtually impossible to prove the absence of a relationship with the same surety that is possible in establishing the presence of one.)

If the evidence is not reasonably convincing either in support of or against causality, the category "inadequate to accept or reject a causal relationship" is used. Evidence that is sparse, conflicting, of weak quality, or merely suggestive—whether toward or away from causality—falls into this category. Under these circumstances, some authors of similar assessments use phrases such as "the evidence does not presently support a causal association." The committee believes, however, that such language does not make the important distinction between evidence indicating that a relationship does not exist (category 3) and evidence that is indeterminate with regard to causality (category 2). The category of "no evidence" is reserved for those cases in which there is a complete absence of clinical or epidemiologic evidence.

The sources of evidence considered by the committee in its assessment of causality include epidemiologic and clinical studies directly addressing the question at hand. That is, the data are specifically related to the effects of the vaccine(s) under review and the adverse health outcome(s) under review—in this report, the MMR vaccine and thimerosal-containing vaccines and the risk of autism.

Epidemiologic studies carry the most weight in a causality assessment. These studies measure health-related exposures and outcomes in a defined set of subjects and use that information to make inferences about the nature and strength of associations between such exposures and outcomes in the overall population from which the study sample was drawn. Epidemiologic studies can be categorized as observational or experimental (clinical trial), and as uncontrolled or controlled. Among these categories, experimental studies generally have the advantage of random assignment to exposures and are therefore the most influential in assessing causality. Uncontrolled observational studies are important but are generally considered less definitive than controlled observational studies. Ecological studies are another category of epidemiological studies that use populations or groups of people, rather than individuals, as the units of analysis (Last et al., 1995). Because the joint distribution of the study factors(s) and disease within each group is unknown in ecological studies, it is difficult to make any causal inferences regarding the association between an exposure and disease at the individual level (Kleinbaum et al., 1982). The committee also separates those studies that analyze data from passive reporting systems into a separate category. Case reports and case series are generally inadequate by themselves to establish causality. Despite the limitations of case reports, the causality argument for at least one vaccine-related adverse event (the relationship between vaccines containing tetanus toxoid and Guillain-Barré syndrome) was strengthened most by a single, well-documented case report on recurrence of the adverse event following readministration of the vaccine, a situation referred to as a "rechallenge" (IOM, 1994a).

Biological Mechanisms

The committee's causality assessments must be guided by an understanding of relevant biological processes. Therefore the committee's scientific assessment includes consideration of biological mechanisms by which immunizations might cause an adverse event. The evidence reviewed comes from human, animal, and *in vitro* studies of biological or pathophysiological processes relevant to the question before the committee. This kind of review was referred to in previous reports of this committee on vaccines and autism (IOM, 2001a,b) and others (IOM, 1991, 1994a) as an assessment of the "biological plausibility" of a causal relationship. The use of "biologic mechanisms" in lieu of "biologic plausibility" was introduced in the committee's third report (IOM, 2002b). The committee shifted its terminology for several reasons. First, an agreed upon hierarchy of evidence required for assessments of biological plausibility does not exist, nor does an associated terminology (Weed and Hursting, 1998).

Second, the committee noted that the term biological plausibility is associated with a particular set of guidelines (sometimes referred to as the Bradford Hill criteria) for causal inference from epidemiological evidence (Hill, 1965). In that context, an assessment of the biological plausibility of an association demonstrated by epidemiological analysis is meant to ensure that such an association is consistent with current biological knowledge. Evidence regarding biological plausibility, however, can never prove causality. It is also meant to guard against attributions of causality to biologically implausible statistical associations that might result from studies that have not adequately accounted for important variables. [1]

Third, the committee understands that some readers of its reports are confused by what might be perceived as contradictory findings. Although the committee has previously stated that biological plausibility can range across a spectrum, readers sometimes regard the term with a degree of certainty or precision the committee never intended. When other evidence of causality is available, biological plausibility adds an additional piece of supportive evidence. However, in the absence of other evidence pointing to a causal relationship, use of the term biological plausibility, as ingrained in the language of causal inference, seems to add confusion.

Thus the committee concluded in its third report (IOM, 2002b) that for future reports, the lack of clarity in the phrase "biological plausibility" warranted the adoption of new terminology and a new approach to its discussion of biological data. The committee decided to review evidence regarding "biological mechanisms" that might be consistent with the proposed relationship between a vaccine exposure and given adverse events.

The biological mechanisms section of the report is written distinct from any argument regarding the causality of such relationships. This is not meant to imply that current understanding of biological processes does not shape or guide assessments of causality. When convincing statistical or clinical evidence of causality is available, biological data add support. This committee, however, is often faced with a set of circumstances in which the epidemiological evidence is judged inadequate to accept or reject a causal association between a vaccine exposure and an adverse event of concern. It is then left with the task of examining proposed or conceivable biological mechanisms that might be operating if an epidemiologically sound association *could* be shown between vaccine exposure and an adverse event. Identification of sound mechanisms could influence the development of an appropriate research agenda and give support to policymakers, as decisions frequently must be made in situations of incomplete information regarding causality. Finally, there is often value in understanding and pursuing possible biological mechanisms even if the epidemiological evidence suggests a

---

[1]For example, although a strong statistical relationship might exist between a woman's risk of breast cancer and the number of bathrooms in her home, there is no mechanism based on knowledge of cancer biology that could indicate the relationship is causal. Rather, the number of bathrooms is associated with socioeconomic status, which is associated with such factors as diet that can be linked mechanistically to cancer biology. The biological implausibility of an association between the number of bathrooms in a house and the risk of breast cancer weakens the argument for a causal relationship. In other cases, a review of the biological plausibility of an association might add reassurance that the epidemiological findings point toward or reflect causality. Occasionally an epidemiological observation has been explained by a reasonable biological mechanism that, on further investigation, appeared not to be relevant for the pathophysiology.

lack of a causal association. New epidemiological studies could lead one to revise a previous causality assessment thus giving sound biological mechanisms more prominence in future assessments. Also, a review of biological data could give support to the negative causality assessment or could cause one to reconsider or pursue the epidemiological findings further. However, absent evidence of a statistical association, or convincing clinical evidence, biological mechanisms cannot be invoked to prove causality.

The committee has established three general categories of evidence on biological mechanisms:

1. *Theoretical.* A reasonable mechanism can be hypothesized that is commensurate with scientific knowledge and does not contradict known physical and biological principles, but has not been demonstrated in whole or in part in humans or animal models. Postulated mechanisms by which a vaccine might cause a specific adverse event but for which no coherent theory exists would not qualify for this category. Thus, "theoretical" is not a default category, but one that requires thoughtful and biologically meaningful suppositions.

2. *Experimental.* A mechanism can be shown to operate in *in vitro* systems, animals, or humans. But experimental evidence often describes mechanisms that represent only a portion of the pathological process required for expression of disease. Showing that multiple portions of a process operate in reasonable experimental models strengthens the case that the mechanisms could possibly result in disease in humans, but it cannot establish proof.

Some experimental evidence is derived under highly contrived conditions. For example, achieving the results of interest may require extensive manipulation of the genetics of an animal system, or *in vivo* or *in vitro* exposures to a vaccine component that are extreme in terms of dose, route, or duration. Other experimental evidence is derived under less contrived conditions. For example, a compelling animal or *in vitro* model might demonstrate a pathologic process analogous to human disease when a vaccine antigen is administered under conditions similar to human use. Experimental evidence can also come from studies in humans. In any case, biological evidence is distinct from the epidemiologic evidence obtained from randomized controlled trials and other population-based studies that are the basis for the causality assessment.

3. *Evidence that the mechanism results in known disease in humans.* For example, a wild-type infection causes the adverse health effect associated with the vaccine, or another vaccine has been demonstrated to cause the same adverse effect by the same or a similar mechanism. Data from population-based studies of the risk of adverse outcomes following vaccination constitute evidence regarding causality, not biological mechanisms.

If the committee identifies evidence of biological mechanisms that could be operating, it offers a summary judgment of that body of evidence as weak, moderate, or strong. Although the committee tends to judge biological evidence in humans as "stronger" than biological evidence from highly contrived animal models or *in vitro* systems, the summary judgment of the strength of the evidence also depends on the quantity (e.g., number of studies or number of subjects in a study) and quality (e.g., the nature of the experimental system or study design) of the evidence. Obviously, the conclusions drawn from this review depend both on the specific data and scientific judgment. To ensure that its own summary judgment is defensible, the committee aims to be as explicit as possible regarding the strengths and limitations of the biological data.

The committee's examination of biological mechanisms reflects its opinion that available information on possible biological explanations for a relationship between immunization and an adverse event should influence the design of epidemiologic studies and analyses. Similarly, the consideration of confounders and effect modifiers is essential in epidemiologic studies and depends on an understanding of the biological phenomena that could underlie or explain the observed statistical relationship. The identification of sound biological mechanisms can also guide the development of an appropriate research agenda and aid policymakers, who frequently must make decisions without having definitive information regarding causality.

In addition, investigating and understanding possible biological mechanisms is often of value even if the available epidemiologic evidence suggests the absence of a causal association. A review of biological data could give support to the negative causality assessment, for example, or it could prompt a reconsideration or further investigation of the epidemiologic findings. If new epidemiologic studies were to question the existing causality assessment, the biological data could gain prominence in the new assessments.

Published and Unpublished Data

Published reports carry the most weight in the committee's assessment because their methods and findings are laid out in enough detail to be assessed. Furthermore, those published works that undergo a rigorous peer review are subject to comment and criticism by the entire scientific community. Thus the committee generally cannot rely heavily on unpublished data in making its scientific assessments (regarding either causality or biological mechanisms) because they usually lack the commentary and criticism provided by peer review and must therefore be interpreted with caution. The committee also relies on editorial and peer-review procedures to ensure the disclosure of potential conflicts of interest that might be related to sources of funding of the research studies. The committee does not itself investigate the sources of funding of the published research reports it reviews, nor do funding sources influence the committee's interpretation of the evidence.

Unpublished data and other reports that have not undergone peer review do have value, however, and are often considered by the committee. They might be used, for example, in support of a body of published, peer-reviewed literature with similar findings. If the committee concluded that the unpublished data were well described, had been obtained using sound methodology, and presented very clear results, the committee could report, with sufficient caveats in the discussion, how the unpublished data fit with the entire body of published literature. Only in extraordinary circumstances, however, could an unpublished study refute a body of published literature.

The Immunization Safety Review Committee's scope of work includes consideration of clinical topics for which high-quality experimental studies are rarely available. Although many other panels making clinical recommendations using evidence-based methods are able to require that randomized trials be available to reach strong conclusions, the IOM committee was convened specifically to assess topics that are of immediate concern yet for which data may just be emerging. Given the unique nature of this project, therefore, the committee deemed it important to review and consider as much information as possible, including unpublished reports. The committee does not perform primary or secondary analyses of unpublished data, however. In reviewing unpublished material, the committee applies generally accepted standards for assessing the quality of scientific evidence, as described above. (All unpublished data reviewed by the committee and cited in this report are available—in the form reviewed by the committee—through the public access files of the National Academies. For a summary of these submissions, see Appendix E. Information about the public access files is available at 202-334-3543 or www.national-academies.org/publicaccess.)

UNDER REVIEW:
VACCINES AND AUTISM

In this report, the committee examines the hypothesis of whether or not the MMR vaccine and the use of vaccines containing the preservative thimerosal can cause autism. The IOM has issued two previous reports examining the role of vaccines in autism. The first report, which reviewed the hypothesized causal association between the MMR vaccine and autism (IOM, 2001a), the committee concluded that the evidence at the time favored rejection of a causal relationship at the population level between MMR vaccine and autism. The committee's conclusion did not exclude the possibility that MMR could contribute to autism in small number of children, given that the epidemiological studies lacked sufficient precision to assess rare occurrences. Thus it was possible that epidemiological studies would not detect a relationship between autism and MMR vaccination in a subset of the population with a genetic predisposition to autism. The biological models for an association between MMR and autism were not established, but nevertheless were not disproved.

In a subsequent report, the committee reviewed the hypothesized link between thimerosal-containing vaccines (TCVs) and a broad range of neurodevelop-mental disorders (NDDs), including autism (IOM, 2001b). In that report, the committee concluded that the evidence was inadequate to accept or reject a causal relationship between exposure to thimerosal from vaccines and the NDDs of autism, attention deficit hyperactivity disorder (ADHD), and speech or lan-guage delay. The committee's causality conclusion was based on the fact that there were no published epidemiological studies examining the potential associa-tion between TCVs and NDDs, and the two unpublished, epidemiological studies that were available (Blaxill, 2001; Verstraeten, 2001) provided only weak and inconclusive evidence of an association between NDDs and TCVs. The com-mittee also concluded that the hypothesis linking TCVs with NDDs was not yet established and rested on incomplete evidence. However, because mercury is a known neurotoxin, and prenatal exposures to methylmercury (a compound closely related to the form of mercury in TCVs) have been documented to negatively affect early childhood development (see NRC, 2000),[2] a potential biological mechanism could be hypothesized based on analogies with this compound.

New epidemiological studies and biological mechanism theories on both issues have emerged since the publication of the two IOM reports. In this report, the committee incorporates the available epidemiological evidence and studies of biological mechanisms relating to vaccines and autism; it does not address the hypothesized link between vaccines and other NDDs.

Autism

Autism is a complex and severe set of developmental disorders characterized by sustained impairments in social interaction, impairments in verbal and non-verbal communication, and stereotypically restricted or repetitive patterns of behaviors and interests (APA, 2000; Filipek et al., 1999; Volkmar and Pauls, 2003). Over time, research has identified subtle differences in the onset and progression of autistic symptoms. Autism is classified under the umbrella cat-egory of "pervasive developmental disorders" (PDDs) (APA, 2000). PDD refers to a continuum of related cognitive and neurobehavioral disorders that reflects the heterogeneity of symptoms and clinical presentations. PDD includes autistic disorder, childhood disintegrative disorder, Asperger's syndrome, Rett's syn-drome, and pervasive developmental disorder not otherwise specified (PDD-NOS, or atypical autism). The term "autistic spectrum disorder" (ASD) has come into common use and is essentially synonymous with the term PDD (Volkmar and

---

[2]For example, there is evidence that fetal exposure to mercury might lead to detectable differ-ences in neurodevelopmental testing that might be consistent with some neurodevelopmental dis-abilities (see NRC, 2000).

Pauls, 2003). In this report, the terms "autism," "autistic," and "autistic spectrum disorders" are used interchangeably to refer to this broader group of pervasive developmental disorders.[3] (See previous IOM report on MMR vaccine and autism (2001a) for a more detailed discussion of the diagnoses under ASD.) Although Rett's syndrome is included among the ASDs, it is considered by many to be a distinct neurologic disorder and thus its diagnosis has not been included in most research evaluating the hypothesized link between vaccines and autism.

Clinical descriptions of ASD suggest two primary types of presentations, including early onset and regression. In the early-onset cases, developmental abnormalities appear within the first year or few months of life, and may be apparent as early as birth. Clinical symptoms of autism can be seen on retrospective, as well as prospective, video analyses by six months of age (Maestro et al., 2002), and on first birthday videos (Osterling and Dawson, 1994), well before the usual age of diagnosis. Most cases of autism appear to be early onset (Bristol et al., 1996); however, the diagnosis is characteristically not made until the second year of life when symptoms become more prominent.

In a second course of autism, suggested by the minority of cases, apparently normal development is followed by regression, or the sudden or insidious loss of previously established developmental milestones, which may exhibit a fluctuating pattern (Rapin, 1997; Tuchman et al., 1991). Estimates of the prevalence of regressive autism are limited and findings are inconsistent (Davidovitch et al., 2000; Hoshino et al., 1987; Kurita, 1985; Lord, 1995; Volkmar, 2001; Werner et al., in press).

Differentiation between these two courses of autism may be confounded by delayed parental recognition of developmental problems that were actually present much earlier in childhood (Mars et al., 1998; Rogers and DiLalla, 1990; Tuchman and Rapin, 1997). Furthermore, it is possible that the regressive form does not represent actual regression of development but rather a failure to progress (Volkmar, 2001). It is an important possibility that regressive autism is a manifestation of a later insult that exacerbates an earlier insult. Because there are conflicting views regarding the frequency and timing of regression, it is the subject of current research efforts.

The consensus of most scientific experts is that autism is generally caused by early prenatal exposures (such as to valproic acid (Moore et al., 2000) or thalidomide (Stromland et al., 1994)) or is linked to early developmental genes (Ingram et al., 2000; Persico et al., 2001; Wassink et al., 2001). Several studies have documented prenatal onset of autism. The neuropathological changes described

---

[3]The term "autistic disorder" refers to a more narrow diagnosis defined by criteria in the *Diagnostic and Statistical Manual of Mental Disorders, 4th edition* (DSM-IV) (APA, 2000).

by Bauman and Kemper (1997) in autopsies of brains of individuals with autism have their origins during the first and second trimesters of gestation, and characteristic arrangements of cellular "minicolumns" described by Casanova et al. (2002) are established by the end of the second trimester. Nelson and colleagues (2001) also identified differences in the neuropeptides and neurotrophins in neonatal blood of children with autism or mental retardation compared to controls. In 99 percent of children in the study with autism and 97 percent of children with mental retardation, concentrations of at least one of the specified neuropeptides and neurotrophins exceeded the concentrations in all control subjects at birth. Courchesne and colleagues (2003) found that the clinical onset of autism was preceded by two phases of growth abnormality, decreased head circumference at birth, and accelerated head growth during the next several years, which argues for altered growth patterns irrespective of specific illnesses, events, or toxicities following birth. In addition, research on twins and families has established a strong genetic component in the etiology of autism (Bailey et al., 1995; Folstein and Rutter, 1977; Steffenburg et al., 1989). High concordance rates are found in monozygotic twins (Bailey et al., 1995; Trottier et al., 1999). Other factors, including infectious, neurological, metabolic, immunological, and environmental insults, may play important roles (Hornig, 2004).

ASDs are indeed heterogeneous, both in their clinical presentations and known biological causes. Historically in the field of autism, once a known cause has been attributed to a subgroup, that diagnosis has been removed from the "spectrum" and is thereafter referred to as a disorder with an "autistic phenotype." Examples include congenital rubella, Fragile X syndrome, tuberous sclerosis, and Rett's syndrome. Among those being evaluated for symptoms of autism for the first time, 5 to 12 percent are attributable to known genetic and medical disorders (Kielinen et al., 2004). It cannot be assumed that the remaining 88 percent of those with "idiopathic autism" are similar with respect to etiology or pathogenesis. While some progress has been made, significant gaps still remain in our understanding of the risk factors and etiological mechanisms of ASD.

Epidemiology of Autistic Spectrum Disorders

There is considerable uncertainty about the prevalence (the proportion of individuals in a population with a given condition) and incidence (the number of new cases in a given population) of autistic disorder and other ASDs and their trends over time. In a recent review (Fombonne, 2002) of 32 studies conducted between 1966 and 2001, the prevalence rates of autistic disorder ranged from 0.7 per 10,000 to 72.6 per 10,000, with a median value of 8.7 per 10,000. After excluding studies with low precision and focusing on recent surveys, the best conservative estimate of the prevalence of autistic disorder is thought to be 10 per 10,000. A separate review of 18 epidemiological studies conducted outside the United States between 1966 and 1997 also concluded that the most reasonable conservative (mean) estimate of the prevalence of autistic disorder is about 10 in 10,000 children (Gillberg and Wing, 1999).[4]

Most of the published literature is uninformative for gauging trends in autism rates (Fombonne, 1999, 2001b). Although recent reviews have concluded that the prevalence of autism has increased over time (Fombonne, 1999, 2002; Gillberg and Wing, 1999), many of the studies examined varied in terms of their diagnostic criteria, case-finding methods, participation rates, precision, and the age and size of the populations studied. Thus it is difficult to discern how much of the observed increase is real or possibly due to other factors, such as the adoption of a broader diagnostic concept of autism, improved recognition of autism, or variations in the precision of the studies (Fombonne, 1999, 2001c; Gillberg and Wing, 1999). Time trends can be evaluated only in studies in which these parameters are held constant.

Historically, few studies have examined the prevalence and incidence of autism in the United States, although more research is emerging in this area. Two studies conducted in the 1980s (Burd et al., 1987; Ritvo et al., 1989a,b) provide similar prevalence estimates of autistic disorder, 3.3 per 10,000 and 3.6 per 10,000, although these rates differ substantially from the prevalence rates found in non-U.S. studies conducted during the same period and those conducted more recently (Gillberg and Wing, 1999).

A more recent epidemiological study conducted by the CDC in Brick Township, New Jersey, found that the estimated prevalence of autistic disorder was 40 per 10,000 (95% CI, 28-56) while the estimated prevalence of ASD was 67 per 10,000 (95% CI, 51-87) (Bertrand et al., 2001). These rates are higher than those reported in previously published studies although, as noted above, there is significant controversy about the actual rate of ASD in the United States. The authors note several factors that may have contributed to the high rates of autism and ASD including: the intensity of case-finding methods, the small size of the target population, the heightened awareness of the issue in the community, and the use of the Autism Diagnostic Observation Schedule-G (ADOS-G) diagnostic tool, which is a sensitive tool that may have led to the inclusion of children with more subtle signs of ASD. Furthermore, the in-migration of families with children having ASD to Brick Township may have led to a clustering of cases in that town and is a possible explanation for the higher rate of autism and ASD found in this study.

Another study by Yeargin-Allsopp and colleagues (2003) estimated the prevalence of ASD in metropolitan Atlanta in 1996 using data from several sources of a population-based developmental disabilities surveillance program.

---

[4]These figures do not include other categories of ASD such as Asperger's syndrome, childhood disintegrative disorder, Rett's syndrome, or atypical autism. Clearly, prevalence estimates would be higher if these categories were included.

They found that the prevalence rate in 3- to 10-year-olds was 34 per 10,000 (95% CI, 32-36). However, the authors noted that they may have underestimated the true prevalence because individuals with autism and other milder cases may have been missed, and younger children may have been too young to be diagnosed. In addition, lower rates in older children may reflect diagnoses made using the narrower DSM-III case definition and the limited number of services for children with autism in the early 1990s.

Two other studies estimated ASD prevalence using state data of individuals receiving services for developmental disabilities. One study (Gurney et al., 2003) estimated that the prevalence of ASD in 6- to 11-year-olds in Minnesota increased from 3 per 10,000 in 1991-1992 to 52 per 10,000 in 2001-2002. However, the authors point out several limitations of their study: diagnostic criteria varied across state districts and over time; and the inability to validate ASD diagnosis and assess the number of children with ASD who were missed or the number of children who had ASD but who did not meet DSM-IV criteria for ASD. A second study (Croen et al., 2002) estimated the prevalence of ASD in eight California birth cohorts using data on the number of children with ASD registered in the California Developmental Services system. From 1987 to 1994, the prevalence was 11 per 10,000 (95% CI, 10.7-11.3), and the prevalence changed from 5.8 per 10,000 in the 1987 birth cohort to 14.9 per 10,000 in the 1994 birth cohort. The authors point out that the prevalence may have been an underestimate resulting from missed diagnoses in the younger children and children with autism not in the Special Education system. Prevalence estimates based on special education data could also be affected by families moving to places where they can obtain better services for children with autism.

A previous report from the California Department of Developmental Services (California Health and Human Services Agency, Department of Developmental Services, 1999) and its revised update (California Department of Developmental Services, 2003), which showed a large increase from 1987 to 2002, has been widely cited as evidence of an increase in the incidence of ASD in the United States. However, the report stresses that the study was not designed to measure trends in autism incidence, and the data should therefore be interpreted with caution. Several methodological limitations have been cited, including the failure to account for changes over time in the population size or composition, in diagnostic concepts, in case definitions, or in age of diagnosis (Fombonne, 2001a).

Thimerosal in Vaccines

Thimerosal, also known as thiomersal, has been used as a preservative in some vaccines and other biological and pharmaceutical products since the 1930s. Thimerosal is an organic mercury compound that is metabolized to ethylmercury and thiosalicylate. FDA regulations require the use of preservatives in multi-dose vials of vaccines, excepting live-virus vaccines, to prevent fungal and bacterial contamination (General Biologics Product Standards, 2000), which can lead to serious illness and death in recipients (Wilson, 1967). Until 1999, thimerosal was contained in over 30 vaccines licensed and marketed in the United States, including some of the vaccines administered to infants for protection against diphtheria, tetanus, pertussis, *Haemophilus influenzae* type b (Hib), and hepatitis B. Prior to 1991, the only TCV that was recommended for all infants was the whole-cell pertussis vaccine (DTP).[5] In 1991, Hib and hepatitis B vaccines were also recommended for all infants (CDC, 1991). Inactivated polio vaccine (IPV) and live viral vaccines, such as measles-mumps-rubella (MMR), varicella, and oral polio vaccine (OPV) do not contain, and have never contained, thimerosal (joint statement of the American Academy of Pediatrics (AAP) and the United States Public Health Service (USPHS), 1999; FDA, 2001).

In addition to its use as a preservative, thimerosal is used as an inactivating or bacteriostatic agent in the manufacturing process for some vaccines. Uses other than as a preservative contribute little to the final concentration of thimerosal in vaccines (Ball et al., 2001). In this report, when the committee refers to thimerosal-free vaccines, it includes vaccines that contain only traces of thimerosal (<0.5 µg Hg per dose) left over from the manufacturing process.

In 1999, FDA determined that under the recommended childhood immunization schedule, infants might be exposed to cumulative doses of ethylmercury that exceed some federal safety guidelines established for ingestion of methylmercury, another form of organic mercury (Ball et al., 2001). Under the 1999 recommended childhood immunization schedule, infants could receive a cumulative dose of mercury from vaccines as high as 187.5 µg during the first 6 months of life, depending on the specific vaccines and administration schedule used. A 2-year-old could receive as much as 237.5 µg of mercury. Also, in 1999, some high-risk children could have received the influenza vaccine, increasing the maximum cumulative dose to approximately 275 µg in the first two years of life (see Table 1).

The maximum cumulative doses of mercury from vaccines in the first 6 months and 2 years of life were then compared to estimated cumulative limits for mercury exposure based on guidelines of the Environmental Protection Agency (EPA), the Agency for Toxic Substance and Disease Registry (ATSDR), the FDA, and the World Health Organization (WHO). This comparison found that 6-month-olds could have received cumulative doses of mercury that exceeded the EPA limits calculated for each body-weight category and that exceeded the ATSDR limits for the lowest-weight infants who also received the influenza vaccine (see Table 2).

In July 1999, the AAP and the USPHS issued a joint statement recommend-

---

[5]Acellular pertussis vaccines (DTaP) replaced whole-cell pertussis (DTP) vaccines on the recommended schedule in the 1990s. Infanrix, the first thimerosal-free DTaP vaccine (produced by Glaxo-Smith Kline) was licensed in 1997 (CDC, 1997).

TABLE 1 Estimated Exposure to Mercury from Vaccines in United States in 1999 and in 2004 (<6 months of age)

Vaccines	1999 Maximum Mercury Dose (μg)	2004 Maximum Mercury Dose (μg)
3 doses of DTaP[†]	75.0	<0.9
3 doses of Hep B[‡]	37.5	<1.5
3 doses of HIB	75.0	0
TOTAL	**187.5**	**<2.4**

Estimated Exposure to Mercury from Vaccines in 1999 and in 2004 (< 2 years of age)

Vaccines	1999 Maximum Mercury Dose (μg)	2004 Maximum Mercury Dose (μg)
4 doses of DTaP[†]	100	<1.2
3 doses of Hep B	37.5	<1.5
4 doses of HIB	100	0
3 doses of influenza*	**[37.5]	**37.5
TOTAL	**237.5 [275]**	**< 40.2**

[†]A trace amount of mercury is present in Tripedia thus, the maximum mercury dose following three doses of Tripedia is <0.9 μg, the maximum mercury dose following four doses of Tripedia is <1.2 μg.
[‡] A trace amount of mercury is present in EngerixB; thus, the maximum mercury dose following three doses of EngerixB is <1.5 μg.
*Children less than 9 years of age receiving the influenza vaccine for the first time are recommended to receive two doses of the vaccine, at least one month apart (CDC, 1999b). A child less than 2 years of age may receive three doses of the influenza vaccine. This could occur if the child turned 6 months of age in October, during the beginning of the influenza season, receives one dose of influenza vaccine then, and subsequently at age 7 months. The child could receive the third dose of influenza vaccine during the following October, at age 18 months.
**ACIP recommended recently that all children 6 to 23 months of age receive the influenza vaccine (CDC, 2004). Previously, the ACIP encouraged influenza vaccination in this age group and recommended vaccination in children with certain risk factors (CDC, 2003a,b). The number in brackets in the 1999 column reflects the amount of mercury if children received the influenza vaccine.
SOURCE: Joint statement of the American Academy of Pediatrics (AAP) and the United States Public Health Service (USPHS), 1999; FDA 2001, 2004e.

ing the removal of thimerosal from vaccines as soon as possible (CDC, 1999b). The statement also recommended that the first dose of hepatitis B vaccine could be postponed (from birth until 2-6 months of age) for infants born to low-risk mothers. With the licensure of a thimerosal-free hepatitis B vaccine in August 1999 and approval of a thimerosal-free preservative hepatitis B vaccine in March 2000, children had access to a hepatitis B vaccine that did not contain thimerosal

TABLE 2 Calculated Exposure Limits for Mercury, Using Various Agency Guidelines for Exposure to Methylmercury, in Infants ≤ 6 Months of Age by Percentile Body Weight

Agency	Percentile Body Weight		
	5th	50th	95th
EPA	**65 µg**	**89 µg**	**106 µg**
ATSDR	**194 µg**	266 µg	319 µg
FDA	259 µg	354 µg	425 µg
WHO	305 µg	417 µg	501 µg

- Calculate Exposure Limit = dose/kg body weight/week × average weight x 26 weeks × 0.932 (mercury molecular weight/methylmercury molecular weight); e.g., EPA calculated exposure limit = 0.7 µg/kg body weight/week × 26 weeks × (2.36kg + 5.25 kg)/2 × 0.932 = 65 µg.
- Assumes average of 5th, 50th, and 95th percentile weight for females at birth (2.36 kg, 3.23 kg, 3.81 kg) and 6 months (5.25 kg, 7.21 kg, 8.73 kg) = 3.81 kg, 5.22 kg, 6.27 kg. Females were selected because their smaller body weight makes them more susceptible than males.
- Recommended limits on methylmercury exposure: EPA: 0.1 µg/kg body weight/day; ATSDR: 0.3 µg/kg body weight/day; FDA: 0.4 µg/kg body weight/day; WHO: 3.3 µg/kg body weight/week. For calculations, daily limits multiplied by 7 to obtain weekly limits.

NOTE: Data were bolded by the IOM, not by the original authors of the table. EPA: Environmental Protection Agency; ATSDR: Agency for Toxic Substances and Disease Registry; FDA: Food and Drug Administration; WHO: World Health Organization.
SOURCE: Ball et al., 2001. Reprinted with permission from *Pediatrics* 107:1150, Table 1, Copyright 2001.

as a preservative by March 2000. With the FDA approval of a second thimerosal-free version of DTaP vaccine in March 2001, all formulations of vaccines on the U.S. recommended childhood immunization schedule for children 6 years of age or younger became available free of thimerosal used as a preservative. Based on information from vaccine manufacturers provided to the FDA, the lots of vaccine manufactured before this time that contained thimerosal as a preservative and had been released to the market had expiration dates in 2002 (FDA, 2004e). Based on these changes, the maximum amount of mercury from vaccines on the recommended childhood immunization schedule that an infant (less than 6 months of age) can now be exposed to is <3 µg,[6] down from 187.5 µg in 1999 (FDA, 2001; 2004e). (See Appendix C for thimerosal content in currently licensed vaccines.)

---

[6] 3 µg is the maximum amount that could have been received by an infant in the first 6 months of life if they received trace-containing formulations (e.g., Engerix B hepatitis B vaccine, Tripedia DTaP vaccine) as opposed to those that contain no thimerosal (e.g., Recombivax HB hepatitis B vaccine pediatric formulation, Infanrix DTaP, Daptacel DTaP) (FDA, 2004d).

MMR Vaccine

The MMR vaccine consists of three separate attenuated viruses directed against three different diseases.[7] The MMR vaccine has been hypothesized many times over the years to cause neurologic disorders, including encephalitis or encephalopathy. A demonstrated biologic mechanism exists for this association, because natural (wild-type) measles clearly infects the central nervous system (CNS) and can lead to clinical neurologic events. In addition, maternal rubella virus is known to produce CNS-related birth defects (Greenberg et al., 1957). Although biologic mechanisms exist for neurologic effects, the totality of biological, clinical, and epidemiological data led previous IOM committees to conclude that the evidence was inadequate to accept or reject a causal relationship between MMR vaccine and encephalopathy, subacute sclerosing panencephalitis (SSPE), or residual seizure disorder (IOM, 1994a).

The controversy regarding the putative link between the MMR vaccine and autism began in 1998 when Dr. Andrew Wakefield and colleagues published a case series describing 12 children with pervasive developmental disorder associated with gastrointestinal (GI) symptoms and developmental regression (Wakefield et al., 1998). For eight of these children, the onset of their behavioral problems was associated, through retrospective accounts by their parents or physicians, with MMR vaccination. This study put forth a hypothesis that a new phenotype of autism characterized by GI symptoms and developmental regression could be associated with the MMR vaccine. While the authors acknowledged that the study did not prove an association between MMR and the conditions seen in these children, the report generated considerable interest and concern about a possible link between MMR vaccination and ASD—regressive autism in particular. A recent statement from 10 of the original 13 authors states that the data were insufficient to establish a causal link between MMR vaccine and autism (Murch et al., 2004).

In response to public concern about the safety of the MMR vaccine following the 1998 study, a number of researchers initiated epidemiological studies to examine the association between ASD and the MMR vaccine. Since the committee's 2001 report, in fact, researchers have published six new epidemiological studies (DeStefano et al., 2004; DeWilde et al., 2001; Madsen et al., 2002; Makela et al., 2002; Takahashi et al., 2003; Taylor et al., 2002), and have conducted research on a number of potential biologic mechanisms. The committee thus reviewed the additional epidemiological evidence and lines of inquiry regarding biological mechanisms that were raised subsequent to its last report and its conclusions are given in the present report.

---

[7]Because MMR is a live-virus vaccine, it does not contain thimerosal.

SCIENTIFIC ASSESSMENT

Causality

To assess the issue of causality, the committee examined epidemiologic evidence regarding the possibility of an association between vaccines—specifically, TCVs and MMR vaccine—and autism.

VAERS Reports

The National Childhood Vaccine Injury Act mandates research to improve the safety of vaccines. In the United States, adverse events following vaccination are monitored through a passive surveillance system known as the Vaccine Adverse Events Reporting System (VAERS) co-administered by the CDC and the FDA. Reports are voluntarily submitted to VAERS by health care providers, vaccinees, manufacturers, and others, and are accepted into VAERS regardless of whether the vaccine plausibly caused the adverse event (Chen, 1994; Singleton et al., 1999; Varricchio, 1998).

VAERS' strengths are its national scope and its potential to detect in a timely manner rare adverse events that were not identified during prelicensure clinical trials (Singleton et al., 1999). The centralized reporting enables detection of events that might otherwise go unnoticed. For instance, VAERS quickly detected cases of intussusception following release of the rotavirus vaccine, which resulted in the voluntary removal of the vaccine from the market. The system can also be used to monitor vaccine lot-specific safety (Varricchio et al., 2004).

While VAERS is useful in detecting some rare adverse events and generating hypotheses, such a passive surveillance system has many limitations. For one thing, it is subject to underreporting and general reporting bias because of its reliance on voluntary reporting. For another, many reports are incomplete; because they are not formal case reports, information is not presented in standardized fashion. Other limitations include inadequate data on the "denominator" (or total population receiving the vaccine), and lack of an unbiased comparison group. Therefore it is usually not possible to determine causal associations between vaccines and adverse events from VAERS reports nor can VAERS be used to calculate incidence or prevalence of an adverse reaction (Varricchio et al., 2004).

From January 1, 1990, through March 1, 2004, VAERS received approximately 167,340 adverse-event reports for all vaccines (FDA, 2004a); 1,348 of those reports included autism as an adverse event following vaccination (FDA, 2004b). Ninety-three percent of reports that listed autism as an adverse event were reported between 1999 and 2004 (FDA, 2004b), much in the same period in which publicity increased regarding the putative links between MMR vaccine and autism and TCVs and autism. Ten of the 1,348 suggest a rechallenge, but only five of these describe a rechallenge followed by autistic symptoms (FDA, 2004c). The other five describe a recurrence of other reactions such as fever and flu-like symptoms (FDA, 2004c). The committee reviewed these reports, but concluded that they were not informative on the issue of causality, given the analytic limitations of VAERS.

Thimerosal-Containing Vaccines and Autism

Controlled Observational Studies

Denmark. Hviid and colleagues (2003) compared rates of autism and other ASDs in Danish children who received TCV with those who received thimerosal-free vaccine. The study was based on data from the Danish Civil Registration System and other national registries, including the Danish Psychiatric Central Register, data from the National Board of Health, and the National Hospital Discharge Register. (The Danish Civil Registration System is a nationwide register that assigns unique identifier codes to new residents and all individuals born in Denmark and stores demographic information for each individual.) This unique identifier is used to link data in the Danish Civil Registration System to individual information stored in other national registries (Madsen et al., 2002).

The whole-cell pertussis vaccine, produced by Denmark's Statens Serum Institut,[8] was the only TCV recommended in the Danish immunization schedule and was in use from 1970 to 1992. The vaccine was replaced with a thimerosal-free version, which was used until January 1997. This vaccine was itself replaced with acellular pertussis vaccine (which never contained thimerosal) and has been in use ever since. Both versions of the whole-cell pertussis vaccine were administered to children at 5 weeks, 9 weeks, and 10 months of age until they were replaced. The first dose of the TCV contained 50 µg of thimerosal (~25 µg EtHg). The second and third doses each contained 100 µg of thimerosal (~50 µg EtHg).

Information on all children born in Denmark between January 1, 1990, and December 31, 1996, was obtained from the Danish Civil Registration System. Information on receipt of the whole-cell pertussis vaccine was obtained from the National Board of Health. Doses received before June 1, 1992, were considered to contain thimerosal, and doses received after June 1, 1992, were deemed thimerosal free. Children who received thimerosal-free vaccine after one or two doses of TCV were classified according to receipt of TCV. The Danish Psychiatric Central Register provided information on cases diagnosed with autism or other

---

[8]Statens Serum Institut is Denmark's national center for preventing and controlling infectious diseases. It is a nonprofit state enterprise and falls under the Danish Ministry of Health and Interior. By law, Statens Serum Institut is mandated to supply vaccines to the national vaccine program, and does so by producing or purchasing vaccines.

ASDs. Autism and ASD cases were ascertained using the ICD-10 coding scheme. From 1991 to 1994, only inpatients were included in the Danish Psychiatric Central Register. Since 1995, both inpatients and outpatients have been included. The National Hospital Discharge Register provided information on other conditions relevant to autism, including tuberous sclerosis, Angelman syndrome, Fragile X syndrome, and congenital rubella. The Danish Civil Registration System and the Danish Medical Birth Registry provided information on possible confounders.

Follow-up was measured using person-time. Follow-up time began at 1 year of age or January 1, 1991 (whichever occurred last) to diagnosis of autism, other ASDs, or other relevant disorders (tuberous sclerosis, Angelman syndrome, Fragile X syndrome, and congenital rubella), death, disappearance, emigration, 11 years of age, or until December 31, 2000 (whichever occurred first). Poisson regression was used to estimate the rate ratios of autism or other ASDs in those receiving thimerosal-containing whole-cell pertussis vaccine to those receiving thimerosal-free whole-cell pertussis vaccine. In addition, the dose-response relationship between TCVs and autism or other ASDs was estimated as the increase in the rate ratio per 25 μg of EtHg.

A total of 467,450 children were born in Denmark between January 1, 1990, and December 31, 1996.[9] Of this total, 446,695 children received at least one dose of whole-cell pertussis vaccine. For the cohort receiving thimerosal-free vaccinations, there were 1,660,159 person-years at risk. For the cohort receiving TCVs, there were 1,220,006 person-years at risk. Altogether, 407 children were diagnosed with autism, of which 303 children had received thimerosal-free vaccine and 104 received TCV. Some 751 children were diagnosed with other ASDs, of which 430 children received thimerosal-free vaccine and 321 children received TCV. The adjusted rate ratio for autism (adjusting for age, calendar period, child's sex, child's place of birth, birth weight, 5-minute Apgar score, gestational age, mother's age at birth of child, and mother's country of birth) was 0.85 (95% CI, 0.60-1.20). The adjusted rate ratio for other autistic spectrum disorders was 1.12 (95% CI, 0.88-1.43). There was no increase in the rate ratio for autism per 25 μg of EtHg (0.98 [95% CI, 0.90-1.06] or in the rate ratio for other ASDs per 25 μg of EtHg (1.03 [95% CI, 0.98-1.09]).

The authors reanalyzed the data to examine the possibility of misclassification bias (by excluding children vaccinated between June 1, 1992, and December 31, 1992), the robustness of the results (by including only children born between 1991 and 1993), and the impact of missing values (by replacing a missing value with the most common value of the variable). The results from the reanalysis were similar to the original findings. The authors noted that the validity and

---

[9]A total of 5,770 were excluded because of death, emigration, disappearance, tuberous sclerosis, Angelman syndrome, or congenital rubella.

completeness of ASDs diagnosed in the Danish Psychiatric Central Register was high. They also mentioned that the diagnoses of other related conditions in the National Hospital Discharge Register may not be complete, but the lack of completeness is unlikely to seriously confound an association between thimerosal content and ASDs. The authors raised another limitation in that the date of diagnosis, not date of symptom onset, was used to calculate incidence rates, but they stated that because the study examines risk factors and not autism incidence, this may not be a problem. Overall, the authors concluded that the results did not demonstrate an association between TCVs and autism and other ASDs, and there was no indication of a dose-response association between autism and the amount of ethylmercury received through thimerosal.

The committee considered the study as having strong internal validity with the findings demonstrating a secular trend increase in autism, even after the removal of thimerosal in the vaccines used in Denmark. The committee identified a few limitations of the study, including its time-series design and the generalizability of the study's findings to the U.S. situation, especially with regard to the different dosing schedule used in Denmark and the relative genetic homogeneity of the Danish population.

Vaccine Safety Datalink (VSD). Verstraeten and colleagues (2003) conducted a retrospective cohort study to examine whether certain NDDs, including autism, are related to exposure to TCVs. Because of the topic of this report, the committee focuses just on the analyses of the autism outcome. The study was based on data from the Vaccine Safety Datalink (VSD), a large-linked database that includes vaccination, clinical, hospital discharge, and demographic data. The VSD, formed as a partnership between CDC and eight health maintenance organizations (HMOs), was initiated in 1991 and covers approximately 2.5 percent of the U.S. population (Verstraeten, 2001).

The study was conducted in two phases. Phase I was designed to screen data for potential associations between exposures to mercury from TCVs and selected neurodevelopmental outcomes, including autism. Phase II was designed to confirm the hypotheses generated in the first phase. The autism outcome was examined only in Phase I.

In Phase I, the study population included children born between January 1992 and December 1998 who were enrolled continuously during their first year of life in either HMO A or HMO B and who received at least two polio vaccinations by 1 year of age. HMO A included outcomes available throughout the study period, and HMO B included data available beginning in January 1995 with follow-up data available through the end of 2000. Excluded from the study were infants born at a weight of <2500 g and infants with diagnoses of congenital or severe perinatal disorders, or born to mothers with serious medical problems of pregnancy. Of the 23,241 infants born in HMO A and 229,285 infants born in

HMO B between 1992 and 1998, 13,337 from HMO A and 110,833 from HMO B met the eligibility criteria for inclusion in the analyses.

For each child, cumulative vaccine-related mercury exposure was calculated at the end of the first, third, and seventh months of life. Exposure estimates were based on the mean ethylmercury content of each vaccine in multidose vials: each vaccine that a child received was assumed to contain the mean amount of thimerosal reported by manufacturers to the FDA. Thus the ethylmercury content per dose of each childhood vaccine was assumed to be as follows: diphtheria-tetanus-pertussis (whole-cell or acellular), 25.0 μg; hepatitis B, 12.5 μg; and *Haemophilus influenzae* type b, 25.0 μg. The level of mercury exposure was categorized in increments of 12.5 μg. The authors also performed analyses in which exposure was modeled as a categorical variable to show the change in risk for each level of exposure and to check the linearity assumption in the analyses examining exposure as a continuous variable. At 3 months, exposure categories were 0-25 μg, 37.5-50 μg, and ≥ 62.5 μg; and at 7 months the exposure levels were 0-75 μg, 87-162.5 μg, and ≥ 175 μg. The outcomes of interest in the study included a range of neurological disorders as defined by specific ICD-9 diagnostic codes. The committee focused on the autism outcome (ICD-9 299.0).

Cox proportional hazard models estimated the risk of autism at each level of mercury exposure. The follow-up time period for each child in HMO A started at the first birthday and ended at the date of diagnoses or last date of follow-up. The follow-up time period for HMO B was either the first birthday or January 1, 1995 (whichever occurred later) to the date of diagnoses or last date of follow-up. For HMO A, the analysis was stratified by sex, year, and birth month. For HMO B, the analysis was stratified by sex, year, birth month, and clinic with most visits. To obtain sufficient power to detect any association, the investigators decided a priori to evaluate the effect of thimerosal exposure on outcomes with 50 or more cases.

For HMO A, there were 21 reports of autism, with a median age of 49 months. Based on a priori considerations, the relative risk for autism was not calculated in the HMO A cohort. For HMO B, a total of 202 children (median age was 44 months) were diagnosed with autism. Computerized diagnosis of autism was verified by reviewing medical charts of 618 children from both HMO A and B. In HMO A, autism diagnosis was confirmed in 92.3 percent of the records reviewed. In HMO B, autism diagnosis was confirmed in 81.3 percent of the records reviewed.

The relative risk of autism by increase of 12.5 μg of Hg exposure from TCVs is shown in Table 3. Relative risks were also calculated for cumulative exposure at 3 and 7 months (using 0-25 μg as a reference dose), and they are shown in Tables 4 and 5. Because no significant associations were found between autism and exposure to TCVs in Phase I, no further analysis was conducted of the possible relationship between autism and TCV in Phase II of the study. Overall, the study's findings showed no association between TCVs and autism.

TABLE 3 Relative Risk of Autism by Increase of 12.5 µg of Mercury Exposure from Thimerosal-containing Vaccines at HMO B

	1 Month Cumulative Mercury, RR (95% CI)	3 Month Cumulative Mercury RR (95% CI)	7 Month Cumulative Mercury RR (95% CI)
Autism	1.16 (0.78-1.71)	1.06 (0.88-1.28)	1.00 (0.90-1.09)

TABLE 4 Relative Risk of Autism by Category of Cumulative Mercury Exposure at 3 Months in HMO B

	Cumulative Hg Exposure 0-25 µg RR	Cumulative Hg Exposure 37.5-50 µg RR (95% CI)	Cumulative Hg Exposure ≥62.5 µg RR (95% CI)	Chi-square, p-Value
Autism	1.00	1.61 (0.77-3.34)	1.38 (0.55-3.48)	1.84, .40

TABLE 5 Relative Risk of Autism by Category of Cumulative Mercury Exposure at 7 Months in HMO B

	Cumulative Hg Exposure 0-75 µg RR	Cumulative Hg Exposure 87-162.5 µg RR (95% CI)	Cumulative Hg Exposure ≥175 µg RR (95% CI)	Chi-square, p-Value
Autism	1.00	0.95 (0.62-1.46)	0.65 (0.27-1.52)	1.08, .58

Additional analyses were conducted to examine other possible study limitations. This included evaluating the effect of the study exclusion criteria—children not continuously enrolled during the first year of life; low-birth-weight (LBW) children; children with congenital or severe perinatal disorders or born to mothers with serious medical problems of pregnancy; and children who received fewer than two polio vaccinations in the first year of life—on the autism results. Although the data were not shown, the authors report that there was no appreciable effect of the exclusion criteria on the autism results. The authors also noted that the confirmation rate between the computerized diagnoses of autism was high for case ascertainment. Some other limitations noted by the authors included possible underreporting of some vaccinations. Other studies (Mullooly et al., 1999) have estimated that 18 percent of hepatitis B virus (HBV) vaccinations may have been missed in HMO A and 2 percent of HBV missed in HMO B. For other vaccinations, 2 percent is estimated to be missed for Hib and DTwP in

HMO B, and 10 percent for DTwP and 9 percent Hib in HMO A. At the committee's meeting, Davis (2004) mentioned plans for a case-control study to examine the possible association between cumulative exposure to thimerosal in vaccines or RhoGAM from the prenatal period up to seven months of age, and autistic disorder.

Several concerns have been raised regarding the findings of the study by Verstraeten and colleagues (2003). The committee examined the published paper by Verstraeten and colleagues (2003), the letters in response (Verstraeten, 2004), and criticisms of the study in detail (SafeMinds, 2000, 2003, 2004a,b,c). Because of the controversy surrounding this study, the committee discusses these concerns, specifically those related to the autism findings, and describes the authors' responses to these allegations in some detail. (Most concerns were addressed by the authors in the published paper [Verstraeten et al., 2003] or at the committee meeting in February [Davis, 2004].)

One overarching concern expressed by some is that the study design and process may have been manipulated in various ways to reach a negative association (SafeMinds, 2000, 2003, 2004a,b,c). In response, Dr. Davis described the chronology of the VSD study and discussed the differences between the preliminary and final results (Davis, 2004), specifically the relative risks of autism showing a positive but nonsignificant association in earlier analyses versus the relative risk showing no association in the final published study. The difference in preliminary results can be attributed to three major reasons: investigators updated datasets with extended follow-up periods, which allowed for additional cases to be identified; they modified exclusion criteria based on scientific input from the IOM report (IOM, 2001b) and CDC and VSD investigators; and they improved adjustments for health-care-seeking behavior. Other reasons cited for the differences were a modification to the time of exposure, and inclusion of additional variables in the model (Davis, 2004).

The committee notes that it is commonplace for large and important studies to be reviewed along the way, with adjustments often made to improve the eventual validity of the results; thus, it finds nothing inherently troubling in the fact that the VSD study underwent this process. The committee also notes that preliminary results are often misleading and can change substantially as methods are adjusted and more cases and controls are assembled. Indeed, the fact that a conference was held to discuss preliminary findings (Simpsonwood Transcript, 2000) would typically be interpreted as an attempt by the researchers and their sponsors to "get it right," given the high level of interest in the findings.

In these kinds of conferences, it is common for participants to speak candidly of strengths and weaknesses in the research that, if taken out of context, may be misleading. The term "bias," for example, has a specific meaning in research that simply refers to ways in which factors may lead to systematic errors in the true effect estimates, where in lay terms "bias" usually refers to a conscious attempt to distort findings. This type of dual-meaning may lead to confusion and an interpretation that has an entirely different meaning than was intended and understood by the participants. The committee examined the justifications for the analytical approaches and changes made during the VSD study process and found that they conformed to standard epidemiological practice.

Other concerns have been raised regarding specific study methods, including choice of inclusion and exclusion criteria, ascertainment of the outcome (autism) and exposure (thimerosal), potential bias due to health-care-seeking behavior, the dose-response relationship between autism and thimerosal exposure, potential confounders, the limitations of automated databases, and other issues (SafeMinds, 2000, 2003, 2004a,b,c). These are each discussed in turn below:

Exclusion Criteria. Concerns about the appropriateness of the exclusion criteria used in the VSD study have been raised, specifically regarding how excluding subjects may have led towards a bias to the null hypothesis—i.e., shifting the estimates of the size of an association between vaccines and autism toward a modest one or none at all. Subjects were excluded if they did not have documentation in the HMO databases of receiving at least two polio vaccines by 1 year of age, and the authors reasoned that the exclusion criteria ensured that subjects were actually users of the HMO. Subjects with congenital or perinatal disorders or who were born to mothers with serious medical problems during pregnancy, and infants with low birth weight (less than 2,500 g) were also excluded because these outcomes are associated with autism and could confound the study's results.

Dr. Davis presented a reanalysis of the HMO B data that examined the effect of the exclusion criteria on the autism risk estimates. Risk estimates were calculated by including subjects who were originally excluded from the analysis. The analysis was based on an earlier cohort from HMO B, which included 150 subjects (about 75 percent of the size of the final cohort). The data were also presented to the committee at their 2001 meeting. Table 6 depicts the unadjusted relative risk estimates by increase of 12.5 µg of ethylmercury based on exclusion criteria. The risk estimates for autism in the final study cohort did not appreciably differ from the risk estimates of groups after removing exclusion criteria. Autism was not examined in the published LBW analysis.

Autism Diagnosis. Concerns about the ascertainment of cases with autism were raised. To assess the validity of the computerized diagnoses, the authors reviewed 120 medical records of autism cases with an ICD-9 diagnosis and found that 81 to 92 percent of the diagnoses were made by either a clinician or behavioral specialist. The relative risks for autism by increase of 12.5 µg of ethylmercury in chart-validated cases were calculated. There was no evidence of an increased risk for autism. See Table 7.

Several concerns were raised about the possibility of misclassification of cases with autism because of the way the age of the child was handled in the

TABLE 6 Effect of Exclusion Criteria, Unadjusted Relative Risk of Autism by Increase of 12.5 µG of Ethylmercury, HMO B (based on earlier analysis)

Autism	0-1 Month	2-3 Month	4-5 Month	6-7 Month	0-7 Month
Final study cohort (n = 150)	0.99	1.08	0.92	0.97	0.98
Excluding no children (n = 215)	0.94	1.14	0.95	1.02	1.03
Not excluding congenital/perinatal (n not reported)	0.95	1.10	0.94	1.01	1.01
Not excluding children who receive fewer than two polio vaccines by one year of age (n = 213)	0.94	1.10	0.94	1.01	1.00
Not excluding children with low birth weight (n = 196)	0.95	1.10	0.94	1.01	1.01

TABLE 7 Unadjusted Relative Risk by Increase of 12.5 µg of Ethylmercury Chart Verified Diagnosis

Autism	0-1 Month	2-3 Month	4-5 Month	6-7 Month	0-7 Month
Cases with chart-verified diagnoses (n = 120)	0.88	1.10	0.94	0.99	1.00

analyses. One issue related to the published study including different age groups and with varying periods of follow-up time for each subject, leading to the possibility that some cases of autism may have been missed with shorter follow-up. In the analysis, the data were adjusted for month and year of birth and time of follow-up. The statistical-analysis technique should therefore take care of this concern. Another related concern was that inclusion of a younger group (who are less likely to be diagnosed with autism) in the study would bias the thimerosal effect toward zero (or in other words, an odds ratio of 1). Adjusting for age would reduce, but not eliminate, this tendency. However, if there were an effect of thimerosal, one still would anticipate a trend of increasing effect with age—that is, increasing odds ratios with age, and each odds ratio exceeding 1.0, albeit with wide confidence intervals. In this study, there was no such association, even in the older age groups.

Another concern was that children at younger ages with early symptoms of autism might be incorrectly diagnosed with other conditions, such as speech or language delay or "misery disorder." The authors attempted to address this by determining the association between thimerosal and neurodevelopmental outcomes and found no consistent significant associations. However, if there are multiple pathways leading to these disorders, it would be difficult to detect the effect of any one cause—unless it occurred with high frequency and the sample size was large—because the tendency of misclassification of outcome is to dilute measures of effect such as the odds ratio.

Thimerosal Exposure. The authors raised the possible misclassification of thimerosal exposure in using data from the VSD. They cited a study by Mullhooly and colleagues (1999) that evaluated the reliability of automated vaccination data in the VSD. In HMO B, 2 percent of TCVs, specifically neonatal HBV and both DTwP and Hib vaccines, may have been missed. This type of misclassification could lead to a bias toward the null hypothesis; however, in view of the small amount of missing data, the effect is likely to be small.

Health-Care-Seeking Behavior. In their published paper, the authors raised a general concern about how care-seeking behavior would affect the study's results. Speech therapy is not covered in HMO B, and the authors suggested that providers may be less likely to screen for speech and language disorders among young children, and that parents may be a more important factor in the ascertainment of these disorders. Thus parents who are more concerned with neurodevelopmental delays may also be more likely to adhere to a timely vaccination schedule, leading to falsely elevated estimates between thimerosal exposure and certain disorders. To address the effect of health-care-seeking behavior on the risk of autism, Dr. Davis presented an analysis to the committee that implicitly adjusted for care-seeking behavior. They limited this analysis to those who had a complete vaccination schedule—that is, similar health-seeking behavior—but were administered DTP separately versus combined. The combined vaccine has less thimerosal. Using data on autism cases from HMO B (n = 150), they calculated the relative risk of autism between those who received DTP separately (DTP and Hib administered separately) versus those who received DTP combined (combined DTP and HIB administered). In terms of a 25 μg difference in exposure, there was no evidence of an increased risk.

Dose-Response Relationship. In Dr. Davis' presentation, the relative risk of autism was plotted against the levels of cumulative ethylmercury exposure from TCVs administered during the first 7 months of life at HMO A and HMO B from 1992 to 1999. The confidence intervals of the relative risks all went through 1. Dr. Davis noted that there is no evidence of dose-response or an increased risk of autism at any particular exposure.

Autism Incidence. Concerns have been raised that the use of VSD under-estimated the true autism incidence because the study only captured those who sought medical attention. It is important to note that the study was designed to examine the relative risk of developing NDD (including autism) at increasing levels of thimerosal exposure, not to examine the incidence of autism and other NDDs.

Other analyses using VSD. In a separate unpublished analysis of the VSD data, Geier and Geier (2004b) examined the relationship between thimerosal-containing DTP vaccines and autism. Children were included if they received four doses of the DTaP vaccine. These inclusion criteria were used to limit the possibility of differences in health-seeking behavior and to ensure that children were old enough to be diagnosed with an NDD. Overall, 28,056 children received thimerosal-free DTaP vaccine and 55,335 children received only thimerosal-containing DTaP vaccines. The authors analyzed both inpatient and outpatient diagnoses, discarded duplicate cases, and only included children with ICD-9 299.0 (autistic disorder) diagnostic code.

An incidence rate was calculated for each cohort, and the relative risk was determined by dividing the incidence rate in the thimerosal-containing DTP cohort by the incidence rate in the thimerosal-free DTP cohort. The authors "determined the attributable risk by subtracting the incidence rate of each condition examined in the cohort that only received thimerosal-containing DTaP vaccine from the incidence rate in the cohort that only received thimerosal-free DTaP vaccine."

To determine statistical significance, the authors used likelihood ratio chi-square and Fisher's exact test. The authors' assumption is that "the number of conditions and the number of children in the cohort receiving thimerosal-containing DTaP are the observed values. In this analysis, the statistical package contained in Simple Interactive Statistical Analysis (SISA) and Fisher's exact were used, and a double-sided p-value < 0.05 was accepted as statistically significant. In addition, p-values were determined."

They report a relative risk for autism of 9.6 (attributable risk $= 3.04$ per 10,000 children, $p < 0.005$). To check for possible biases, the authors examined the hypersensitivity diagnosis (ICD-9 995.2). They assumed that because of a correlation between hypersensitivity and thimerosal, children who received thimerosal-containing DTaP would have a higher incidence of hypersensitivity. They found a hypersensitivity relative risk of 1.8 (attributable risk $= 26$ per 10,000 children, $p < 0.0001$) when comparing the risk between children who received thimerosal-containing DTaP and those who received thimerosal-free DTaP. "An overall sampling of diagnoses made in the thimerosal-containing DTaP vaccine cohort in comparison to the thimerosal-free DTaP vaccine cohort was designed to determine whether there were significant differences in the health-care-seeking behaviors of children in the vaccine cohorts, because such a difference could account for significant differences in diagnoses within each cohort examined." The relative risk for health-care-seeking behavior in those who received thimerosal-containing DTaP vaccine was 0.77 (p < 0.0001).

Dr. Geier and Mr. Geier presented to the committee an unpublished analysis of the VSD data. Only one slide depicted this information, and it demonstrated an increasing relationship between autism relative risk and amount of thimerosal. The basis of this calculation was not provided and additional data and methods were not described. Overall, the committee found the results of their analyses using VSD data uninterpretable, primarily due to the lack of a complete description of their methods, specifically in how they determined whether individuals belonged to the unexposed or exposed group. Given this lack of clarity, it is unclear how the incidence rate and the estimate of the relative risk could be calculated. The committee finds the results uninterpretable and, as such, non-contributory with respect to causality.

Other Issues. Verstraeten and colleagues (2003) discussed in their paper general limitations of analyzing VSD data. For example, they were unable to control completely for other potential confounding factors. In HMO B, the clinic that a child attended may have acted as a confounder. Also, the HMO databases did not provide information on other possible confounders, such as maternal smoking, lead exposure, or fish consumption. The authors noted, however, that it is unclear how these variables relate to the child's vaccination status and thereby confound the results.

The authors also cited several limitations when using automated databases, particularly the inability to separate the effects of thimerosal from other vaccine ingredients. The authors conducted a subanalysis by comparing risks associated with DTwP or DTaP vaccine and Hib vaccine given separately or combined. The thimerosal content of these vaccines differed in that the combined vaccine contained 25 μg of Hg and the two vaccines administered separately totaled 50 μg of Hg. There was no difference in estimates of speech or language delays (speech delay RR = 1.04 [95% CI, 0.85-1.27]; language delay RR = 1.29 [95% CI, 0.91-1.82]). There was a significant decreased risk for attention deficit disorder (ADD) (RR = 0.70 [95% CI, 0.52-0.95]).

In summary, the VSD study has several strengths and limitations. Strengths of the study include the following: vaccine information was available on the individual level, a subset of autism diagnoses were validated by medical record review, related diagnoses were examined to address possible misclassification, and a sensitivity analysis was conducted to determine the effect of exclusion criteria on study results. Limitations include the study's ability to answer whether thimerosal in vaccines causes autism because the study tests a dose-response gradient, not exposure versus non-exposure. Also, the small number of cases and instability of some of the risk estimates may affect the findings. Given these strengths and limitations, and with the effect estimates, although nonsignificant, near or below 1, the study showed no association between TCVs and autism.

Ecological Studies

Denmark. Madsen and colleagues (2003) conducted an ecological study comparing the trend in autism incidence in Denmark to the use of TCVs in Denmark from 1971 to 2000.

All together, TCVs were used in Denmark from 1961 to 1992. From 1961 to 1970, only DTP vaccines contained thimerosal, and children received four doses at 5, 6, 7, and 15 months of age. From 1970 to 1992, only whole-cell pertussis vaccine contained thimerosal, and children received three doses at 5 and 9 weeks of age and again at 10 months of age. Each dose of the vaccine contained 0.01 percent thimerosal, or 50 μg ethylmercury, except for the first dose of the whole-cell pertussis vaccine, which contained 25 μg of ethylmercury per mL of vaccine. From 1961 to 1970, by the age of 15 months, children received a total of 400 μg of thimerosal, or 200 μg of ethylmercury. From 1970 to 1992, children received a total of 250 μg of thimerosal, or 125 μg of ethylmercury, by 10 months of age.

Autism cases were obtained from the Danish Psychiatric Central Research Register, a national register that includes all psychiatric admissions. The register included only inpatient treatments between 1969 and 1995, but added outpatient treatments in 1995. Autism cases diagnosed between January 1, 1971, and December 31, 2000, in children 2 to 10 years of age were included in the analysis. Diagnoses were psychosis proto-infantilis (ICD-8 299.00), psychosis infantilis posterior (ICD-8 299.01), infantile autism (ICD-10 F84.0), or atypical autism (ICD-10 F84.1).

Autism incidence rates were calculated by age group for each year between 1971 and 2000. Incidence was calculated as the number of children by age and year and diagnosed for the first time divided by the total number of people living in the Denmark at that same age and year. A total of 956 children were diagnosed with autism. Overall, the incidence rate remained level until 1990, then increased and peaked in 1999, and subsequently decreased.

Because autism rates continued to increase after the elimination of TCVs in Denmark, the authors concluded that the results of the study did not support a correlation between thimerosal in vaccines and autism incidence. The authors raised a concern, however, about the effect of adding outpatients to the Danish Psychiatric Central Research Register on the trends in autism incidence. A reanalysis was conducted, limiting itself to inpatient data only, and the authors found similar trends in autism rates, although the data were not shown. However, despite the reanalysis the authors stated that autism incidence after 1995 may have been exaggerated due to the change in including outpatient cases into the Danish Psychiatric Central Register. This limits the study's contribution to causality.

Denmark. Stehr-Green and colleagues (2003) also conducted an ecological study that compared the number of autism cases per year to the use of TCV in Denmark and Sweden. The data on Sweden are described below. The Danish Statens Serum Institut provided information on the use of TCVs in Denmark. From 1970 to 1989 only whole-cell pertussis vaccines contained thimerosal. By April 1992, the production of whole-cell pertussis ceased and by the end of 1992, its use was eliminated entirely in Denmark.

The number of autism cases was obtained from the Danish National Centre for Register-Based Research, which includes both outpatient and inpatient information on children diagnosed with neurological disorders. Children in the registry included those admitted to a psychiatric hospital or who received outpatient care prior to 1994 with a diagnosis of psychosis proto-infantilis (ICD-8 299.00) or psychosis infantilis posterior (ICD 299.01) and, after 1994, those diagnosed with infantile autism (ICD-10 F84.0) or atypical autism (ICD-10, F84.1). The number of 2- to 10-year-olds diagnosed with autism was totaled for each year between 1983 and 2000.

The number of autism cases among 2- to 10-year-olds remained level before 1990, at less than 10 cases per year, but the number of cases peaked in 1999 to 181. By the end of 2000, there was an estimated autism prevalence of 8.1 cases per 10,000 persons. In contrast, the proportion of children receiving 125 μg of ethylmercury from three doses of whole-cell pertussis vaccine by 10 months of age remained level between 1970 and 1991, but decreased from 1991 to 1993 as thimerosal was eliminated from whole-cell pertussis vaccines. Based on these results, the authors concluded that the results did not support the hypothesis that TCVs are responsible for increasing autism rates. Possible reasons for the autism increase may be due to the changes in the inclusion criteria in the national register, diagnostic changes (from ICD-8 diagnostic coding to ICD-10), and the fact that, prior to 1992, cases diagnosed in one large clinic (about 20 percent of all cases in Sweden) were not included. The ecological nature of the study limits the study's contribution to causality.

Sweden. Stehr-Green and colleagues (2003) conducted an ecological study that examined autism data from Denmark and Sweden. The data from Denmark are described above. In Sweden, autism information was collected on the national level. Cases were inpatients diagnosed between 2 and 10 years of age and diagnosed with either infantile autism or atypical autism (ICD-9 299.x from 1987 to 1997; ICD-10 F84.x from 1997 to 1999). Incidence was calculated by dividing the number of autism cases diagnosed among these inpatients by the total number of person-years accumulated during the time period (multiplied by 100,000 person-years). The result was that autism increased in the mid- to late 1980s and rose from a rate of 5-6 cases per 100,000 person-years before 1985 to 9.2 cases per 100,000 person-years in 1993.

The Swedish Institute for Infectious Disease Control provided information on the time period of use and vaccine-specific amounts of thimerosal for all vaccines used in Sweden. Recommended vaccines that contained thimerosal included DTP vaccine, which was replaced by a thimerosal-free vaccine in 1979, and diphtheria-tetanus vaccine, which was used until 1992. Vaccines contained 0.01 percent thimerosal. Other children may have been exposed to thimerosal-containing Hib vaccine or acellular pertussis vaccines, used in clinical trials prior to 1992. Since 1992, however, thimerosal has not been included in recommended childhood immunizations. Still, hepatitis B vaccine containing thimerosal may have been given to a small number of children who were born to high-risk mothers. Overall, most children in Sweden, prior to 1992, received two doses of DTP or DT and were estimated to have a cumulative dose of ethylmercury of 75 µg by 2 years of age.

The authors concluded that the study did not demonstrate a correlation between thimerosal in vaccines and autism rates because autism rates in Sweden continued to increase after the elimination of thimerosal from vaccines. The authors noted that the data only reflected cases diagnosed in inpatient settings and that the increase in autism may result from changes in diagnostic criteria and increasing awareness of autism and related disorders. The ecological nature of the study limits the study's contribution to causality.

United States. Geier and Geier (2004a)[10] examine the hypothesized association between exposure to TCVs and autism using data on distributed vaccine doses from the CDC's Biologic Surveillance Summaries[11] (BSS) and caseloads of children with autism who were enrolled in special education programs from the U.S. Department of Education (DOE) reports. Autism cases were based on the DOE's definition of autism and data collection standards.[12,13] The authors

---

[10]We classified this study as an ecological study because it relies on aggregate data rather than individual-level data to make inferences about causality. However, the authors appear to attempt an individual-level analysis by assuming thimerosal exposure for each child in the birth cohorts, but it is unclear how this can be given the data they used. Based on the available information, the study design is indeterminate.

[11]The CDC's BSS receives voluntary reports from all manufacturers of distributed and returned vaccine doses (Rosenthal et al., 1996).

[12]Every year, the DOE prepares a report for Congress, as mandated by the Individuals with Disabilities Education Act (IDEA), the federal law that supports special education and related services for children and youth with disabilities. The report contains information about many aspects of the IDEA program, including characteristics of the students served, programs and services, and policies. Data have been collected since 1976. Early data were collected by age group rather than by individual age year. Autism was added as a disability category per the 1990 amendments to IDEA. Autism was an optional disability category for federal reporting for 1991-1992 and became a required category in 1992-1993. Prior to the introduction of autism category in 1990, IDEA served students with autism, but for reporting purposes they were included in a different disability category. (Online. Available at: http://www.ideadata.org/docs/bfactsheetcc. doc.)

[13]The number of autism cases in the special educational system was obtained from the 1999, 2000, and 2003 DOE reports.

estimated the number of children who developed autism for the birth cohorts in each of the following years: 1981-1985 and 1990-1996. The authors estimate the prevalence of autism in each cohort by dividing the number of estimated cases of autism in each birth cohort by the number of live births in that cohort, using data from CDC's annual live birth surveillance data. The authors assumed an average mercury exposure for each child in the birth cohorts based on the aggregate number of doses of TCV[14] distributed per the CDC's Biologic Surveillance Summary,[15] and on the aggregate number of births in that cohort. (Because the BSS only provides aggregate data on doses distributed, it is not possible to determine individual-level exposures. See discussion below.)

They plotted the prevalence of autism for each birth cohort against the assumed average mercury dose that children received in each birth cohort. They reported a slope of 1.6 and a linear regression coefficient of 0.94.[16] The authors note that the prevalence of autism increased sixfold from approximately 50 cases per 100,000 to approximately 300 cases per 100,000.

Using the 1984 cohort as a baseline, they also compared the prevalence of autism and additional mercury doses that children received from childhood vaccines in the 1984 cohort to that of other birth cohorts (1985 and 1990-1996). They calculated odds ratios (95% CI) for each successive birth cohort in comparison to the 1984 cohort. They plotted the odds ratios (95% CI) in comparison to the assumed average increased mercury doses from TCVs based upon a 1984 baseline-birth cohort. They reported "a statistically increased odds ratio" for the prevalence of autism compared to the 1984 baseline-birth cohort, and "each statistically significant odds ratio correlated with increasing mercury doses that children received from thimerosal-containing childhood vaccines" (p. 134). They report the slope of the line in this figure was 0.023 and the linear regression coefficient was 0.89. While the ORs and CIs were depicted graphically, specific results and calculations were not provided in the paper.

In a second paper, Geier and Geier (2003a)[17] compared the number of speci-

---

[14]In this analysis, TCVs included DTwP, DTaP, DTwPHib, DTaPHib, Hib, and pediatric hepatitis B. They determined the amount of mercury in each vaccine based on information from a previous IOM report (IOM, 2001b).

[15]They used the number of pediatric hepatitis B vaccines distributed by SmithKline and the total number of heptatis B vaccines distributed by Merck (Merck did not distinguish between pediatric and adult doses) to estimate hepatitis B doses administered.

[16]The authors appear to use the term "linear regression coefficient" in their analyses to refer to the coefficient of determination (R-sq), although these are distinct concepts. Slope (or partial slope) and coefficient are generally interchangeable terms in the context of regression. Data and variables used in these regression models were not included.

[17]We also classified this study as an ecological study because it relies on aggregate data rather than individual-level data to make inferences about causality. However, the authors appear to attempt an individual-level analysis by assuming thimerosal exposure for each child in the birth cohorts, but it is unclear how this can be given the data they used. Based on the available information, the study design is indeterminate.

fied disabilities reported over time in the DOE data to the estimated doses of mercury children received using data from the BSS. The DOE disability categories that were examined included autism, speech disorders, orthopedic impairments, visual impairments, and deaf-blindness. The prevalence of each of these outcomes was calculated for specific birth cohorts (each of the years 1984-1985 and 1990-1994) by dividing the number of each reported outcome by the number of births for each birth cohort (using CDC's surveillance data). Using data on annual distributed vaccine doses from the BSS, they estimated the average amount of mercury each child received in a birth cohort, although there is no way to determine individual exposures from these data. When the prevalence of autism and other outcomes were plotted against the amount of mercury each child received, the results depicted a positive trend. They report that the OR of autism increased by 0.014 µg of mercury and that the overall OR of autism was 2.5.

These studies are characterized by serious methodological problems. First, the DOE dataset that they use as the basis for the autism prevalence estimates has significant limitations. These data are based on children with a diagnosis of autism who receive special education services, which may or may not reflect the true prevalence of autism. Additionally, the child count is a cross-sectional (i.e., point-in-time) count of students served. The appropriateness of the transformation of the cross-sectional autism-caseload data into birth-cohort prevalence data, as was done in their studies, is questionable. Transforming the cross-sectional data by dividing by birth cohort creates the artificial impression of a cohort effect when the data are cross-sectional in nature (Fombonne, 2001a). Furthermore, changes in either states' policies or IDEA's reporting practices can affect the caseload numbers from year to year. For instance, autism caseload may vary from year to year as the result of policy changes, such as changes to the states' eligibility criteria for particular disabilities. (There is no federal standard for eligibility; states have varying criteria for eligibility). Similarly, prior to the addition of the autism category in 1990, IDEA served students with autism, but for reporting purposes they were reported in a different disability category (see http://www.ideadata.org/docs/bfactsheetcc.doc). The addition of the autism category in 1990-1991 may have led to a significant increase in the number of children reported because of the availability of services. These limitations can bias the autism prevalence estimates and make it very difficult to interpret trends over time.

One of the fundamental flaws is that the papers do not clearly delineate the unit of analysis (individual vs. group) nor do they explain how individuals are allotted into exposed and unexposed groups or how groups-level rates are constructed. It is not possible to assess individual mercury exposure using data from the BSS. The BSS provides information on the number of distributed vaccine doses rather than the number of doses administered. It is unknown whether all the vaccines that were distributed were administered in a given year, or whether the vaccines that were administered were given to separate individuals or given in multiple doses. Furthermore, the BSS does not provide information about the distribution of vaccines by age group or birth cohort (Varricchio et al., 2004). In other words, the number of vaccines distributed in 1984 may not be the same number of doses received by children born that year.

Finally, the description of analytical methods was not transparent and important details were omitted. For example, regression models were not specified, the frequency distribution of variables was not provided, and actual calculations of statistics were not clear or not reported. As a result of these limitations, the committee found these studies to be uninterpretable and, therefore, noncontributory with respect to causality.

Studies of Passive Reporting Data

United States. Geier and Geier conducted three similar studies (Geier and Geier, 2003a,b,d) to investigate the role of thimerosal-containing DTP vaccine with autism and other adverse outcomes. These studies compare the frequency over time of reported adverse events assumedly associated with administered doses of thimerosal-containing DTP vaccine versus the frequency of reported adverse events assumedly associated with administered doses of thimerosal-free DTP vaccine. They hypothesized that the DTP vaccine, whether containing thimerosal or not, should have a similar incidence rate of adverse events over time.

In each of these studies, data on adverse events were obtained from the descriptions in the VAERS database. The authors also analyzed several control outcomes, defined as "adverse events that were not biologically plausible [sic] linked with thimerosal" (Geier and Geier, 2004b), using data from VAERS. Information from the CDC BSS, which receives voluntary reports from all manufacturers of distributed and returned vaccine doses (Rosenthal et al., 1996), was also used as a proxy for the number of DTP vaccine doses administered in a year.

In the first study (Geier and Geier, 2003d), the authors examine two neurodevelopmental outcomes, autism and speech disorders. Information on the adverse event was obtained from VAERS. They estimated the number of administered doses of thimerosal-containing DTaP and DTwP vaccines from 1992 to 2000, and doses of thimerosal-free DTaP from 1997 to 2000 using data from the BSS. They estimated the number of each adverse event for two groups of individuals: those who assumedly received an average of 37.5 µg of mercury and those who assumedly received an average of 87.5 µg of mercury. They do not explain how they categorized individuals into the two exposure groups, nor is it clear how they could.

They then calculate incidence rate[18] of the adverse events following vaccination. Relative risks were calculated by dividing the incidence rate of a particular adverse event following administration of TCV (DTaP or DTwP) by the incidence rate of a particular adverse event following thimerosal-free (DTaP) vaccine. Relative risks were calculated for the 37.5 μg and the 87.5 μg mercury exposure groups. The relative risks were then plotted against the amount of mercury each child assumedly received. The authors assumed a baseline mercury exposure of zero with a relative risk of 1. The relative risk estimates were graphically depicted in a plot, but were not reported. An R-square was calculated to estimate the association between each adverse event and mercury exposure. The R-squared calculation in the analysis comparing thimerosal-containing DTaP vaccine with thimerosal-free DTaP vaccine was 0.99 for autism. They also report a R-squared of 0.99 for autism in the analysis comparing thimerosal-containing DTwP with thimerosal-free DTaP. The regression models and other calculations were not specified in the paper. The authors concluded that "the analyses showed increasing relative risks for neurodevelop-ment disorders with increasing doses of mercury." In an unpublished paper submitted to the committee (Geier and Geier, 2004b), they also state that this study found "consistent increasing risk dose-response relationships for autism following both of our thimerosal-containing vaccines in our comparison to our thimerosal-free DTaP vaccines." In addition, they report that the control adverse events did not follow an increasing risk dose-response relationship with additional doses of mercury from TCVs.

In a second paper (Geier and Geier, 2003a), the authors conduct a very similar analysis using slightly different outcomes and time period for estimates of administered doses. In this study, they examine several adverse event outcomes from VAERS, including autism, personality disorder, and mental retardation. Control outcomes included febrile seizures, fevers, pain, edema, and vomiting. They estimated the number of administered doses of thimerosal-containing DTaP and DTwP and thimerosal-free DTaP from 1997 to 2001. Reports of adverse events were again categorized as either following an average exposure of 37.5 μg of mercury or an average exposure of 87.5 μg of mercury, but again no information was provided on how these averages and the exposure groups were derived.

The authors calculated ORs by comparing the incidence rate of a particular adverse event following DTP TCV with the incidence rate of a particular adverse

---

[18]The authors have used the epidemiologic measure "incidence rate" incorrectly in this study and in their subsequent studies. An incidence rate is the number of new cases occurring in a defined time period among the population at risk. VAERS cannot be used to calculate incidence rates because the VAERS database does not have complete reporting of all adverse events and because many report events lack a confirmed diagnosis or confirmed attribution to vaccine (Varricchio et al., 2004). Therefore, the numerator for an incidence rate, the number of new events, is incomplete. Further, VAERS does not provide the denominator, that is the population at risk of the event or, in this case, the number of persons vaccinated with the vaccine of interest in the same time period.

event following DTP thimerosal-free vaccine. ORs were calculated for the 37.5 μg and the 87.5 μg mercury exposure groups. The ORs were then plotted against the assumed average amount of mercury received. The authors assumed a baseline exposure of zero with a relative risk of 1. A linear regression coefficient and slopes[19] were reported for each adverse event. The regression model was not described in the paper.

They reported an overall OR for autism of 2.6 and that the OR of autism increased by 0.029 per μg of mercury. Standard errors were graphically depicted in a plot, but were not reported. They reported an R-squared of 0.98 for autism in the analysis comparing thimerosal-containing DTaP with thimerosal-free DTaP. The authors concluded that "the dose-response curves show that increases in odds ratios of neurodevelopmental disorders from VAERS . . . [were] closely linearly correlated with increasing doses of mercury from thimerosal-containing child-hood vaccines and that for the overall odds ratios examined statistical significance was achieved" (p. 100).

In a third paper, Geier and Geier (2003c) conduct the same analysis using data again from the BSS to estimate the administered doses of thimerosal-containing DTaP vaccine from 1992 to 2000 and administered doses of thimerosal-free DTaP vaccines from 1997 to 2000. Outcomes examined were autism, mental retardation, and speech disorder. Control outcomes included deaths, seizures, vasculitis, emergency department visits, total reactive reports, and gastroenteritis.

The authors state that 6,575 adverse events reports after thimerosal-containing DTaP vaccines and 1,516 adverse events reports after thimerosal-free DTaP vaccines were reported in the VAERS database. Relative risks were calculated by dividing the incidence rate of a particular adverse event following DTP thimerosal containing vaccine by the incidence rate of a particular adverse event following DTP thimerosal-free vaccine. Other risk estimates included attributable risk,[20]

---

[19]It appears that the authors use the term "linear regression coefficient" to refer instead to the coefficient of determination (R-sq), although these are distinct concepts. Slope (or partial slope) and coefficient are generally interchangeable terms in the context of regression.

[20]The authors used the epidemiologic measure "attributable risk" incorrectly. As noted by Mann (2003), attributable risk is intended to be a measure of the absolute, rather than the relative, difference in risk among the exposed and unexposed groups. Attributable risk percent, known also as the attributable fraction for the exposed or the etiologic fraction, is defined as (risk among the exposed − risk among the unexposed)/(risk among the exposed) and is mathematically equivalent to (RR−1)/RR × 100. Attributable risk percent is interpreted as the proportion of exposed cases whose disease can be attributed to exposure. A second related concept is the population attributable risk percent (also known as attributable fraction for the population) and is defined as (risk in the population − risk for the unexposed)/(risk in the population). Mathematically equivalent formulas are: (prevalence of exposure among cases) × (RR−1)/RR and (prevalence of exposure in the population) × (RR−1)/(1 + prevalence of exposure in the population) × (RR−1). Geier and Geier (2003a,b,c) calculate attributable risk by subtracting 1 from the relative risk value (RR−1 = attributable risk). Making attributable risk a fraction of the relative risk provides no information on the absolute or actual risk of thimerosal, nor does it provide information on the proportions of disease either among the exposed or population that can be attributed to exposure.

TABLE 8 Risk Estimates and Statistical Significance Testing in Geier and Geier 2003b

Outcome of Interest	Relative Risk	Attributable Risk	Percent Association	Statistical Significance
Autism	6.0	5.0	86	p < 0.05
Mental Retardation	6.1	5.1	86	p < 0.002
Speech Disorders	2.2	1.2	69	p < 0.05

Control Outcome	Relative Risk	Attributable Risk	Percent Association	Statistical Significance
Deaths	1.0	0	50	Not reported
Vasculitis	1.2	0.2	54	Not reported
Seizures	1.6	0.6	61	Not reported
ED Visits	1.4	0.4	58	Not reported
Total reaction reports	1.4	0.4	58	Not reported
Gastroenteritis	1.1	0.1	52	Not reported

which was calculated by subtracting one from the relative risk, and percent association,[21] which was calculated by dividing the relative risk by the relative risk plus 1 and multiplying this sum by 100. Statistical significance was calculated using Fisher's exact test. A p-value of 0.05 was considered significant. The authors provided these estimates and the statistical significance in their paper (see Table 8), and concluded that "an association between neurodevelopmental disorders and thimerosal-containing DTaP vaccines was found."

These three studies have serious methodological limitations that make their results uninterpretable. A major problem with these studies is that they rely on analyses of VAERS data to draw conclusions about causality. VAERS is a passive reporting system that accepts voluntary reports from health care providers, vaccine recipients, manufacturers, and others regarding potential adverse events. Adverse event reports are not formal case reports, but rather are descriptions of symptoms that are temporally associated with receipt of a vaccine or vaccines. All adverse event reports are accepted into VAERS regardless of whether the vaccine plausibly caused the adverse event. VAERS has inherent limitations that include variability in reporting standards, reporting bias (e.g., due to other factors such as media attention), unconfirmed diagnoses, lack of information on people who were immunized but did not report an adverse event, lack of an unbiased comparison group, and variable and potentially significant underreporting of adverse events. While VAERS is useful in generating hypotheses, further validation and studies are required before conclusions on causality can be drawn (Varricchio, 2004).

---

[21]Percent association, which the authors define as [RR/{RR+1} ×100], is not a recognized epidemiologic measure.

In addition, the methods they use to analyze VAERS data, which they state follow methods developed by CDC and FDA (Rosenthal et al., 1996), in fact differ in important ways from methods used by the agencies. Rosenthal et al. (1996) evaluated the safety of acellular pertussis vaccine versus whole-cell pertussis vaccine using VAERS data. They calculated the number of doses distributed for each birth cohort using data from the National Health Interview Survey to obtain immunization coverage in children. These data provided information on age and dose-specific vaccination rates. In addition, the authors adjusted the administered doses for seasonal effects by using data from the VSD vaccination records. By contrast, the Geiers' papers do not make these adjustments, thus limiting the utility of the BSS data on doses administered. In addition, the Geiers' studies do not define a specific time period of interest; and they do not define a period of symptom onset (that is, it is unclear if autism or some other adverse event occurred after receipt of the vaccine) or the time period between vaccine receipt and autism diagnosis.

These studies also do not clearly delineate the unit of analysis (individual vs. group) nor do they explain how individuals are allotted into exposed and unexposed groups or how groups-level rates are constructed. They also make significant assumptions about individuals' vaccine histories, which cannot be accurately known from the VAERS or BSS data, introducing an unknown bias to their results.

The articles also lack a complete and transparent description of their methods and underlying data, making it difficult to confirm or evaluate their findings. That is, no information was provided on specification of regression models, the frequency distribution of variables was not provided, and calculations of statistics were not clear or were not reported. Furthermore, as noted when the measures appear in the text, the epidemiological measures "incidence rate," "relative risk," and "attributable risk" are applied incorrectly in these studies.

The results of their studies are likewise improbable. For instance, in one study (Geier and Geier, 2003a), the R^2 was 0.98, suggesting that the thimerosal content of DTP vaccines (excluding all other TCVs) explains 98 percent of the variation in autism rates. The R^2 is improbably high and means that all other potential factors (e.g., genetic or environmental factors) only explain 2 percent of the variance in autism rates. Furthermore, the R^2 explains variation at the individual level; the authors' calculations, however, are a line through averages. Using averages instead of individual points results in the disappearance of most of the variability in a data set (Nordin, 2004). As a result of these significant methodological limitations, the committee finds the results of their studies to be uninterpretable and, as such, they are noncontributory with respect to causality.

Unpublished Controlled Observational Study

United Kingdom. Miller (2004) presented to the committee a cohort study that examined whether certain NDDs, including autism, are related to exposure to

TCVs. Regarding this study, forthcoming in the journal *Pediatrics*, the committee focused only on the analyses examining the autism outcome. The study was based on data from the U.K.'s General Practice Research Database (GPRD), which is similar to the U.S. VSD; About 500 general practices in the United Kingdom contribute data to the GPRD, which is about 5.7 percent of the population. The study's data cover 1988 to 1999 and include patient consultations, referrals, and vaccine information.

The only TCVs administered routinely to children in the United Kingdom are DTP and DT-containing vaccines. These vaccines contain 50 μg of thimerosal (25 μg of ethylmercury). Since 1990-1991, children have received doses of the vaccine at 2, 3, and 4 months of age (and at 3, 5, and 10 months of age before then). With the 2-3-4 month schedule, children could have received a maximum of 50 μg of mercury at 3 months of age and 75 μg of mercury at 4 and 6 months of age. This amount is less than the maximum amount received by U.S. children. U.S. children could have received 75 μg of mercury after 3 months, 125 μg after 4 months, and 187.5 μg after 6 months. Most children in the United Kingdom receive their vaccines in a timely manner.

Children were included into the study, based on the following criteria: born between 1988 and 1997 into a GPRD practice, enrolled in a GPRD practice for at least 2 years, exact birth data available, and data met "up to standard" criteria of GPRD. A total of 107,152 children were in this cohort, but children were further excluded if their records had data errors, for example, if the vaccination date was prior to the birth date. To reduce the possibility of confounding, individuals with the following conditions were excluded: various congenital, prenatal, perinatal conditions; postnatal conditions during the first 6 months; or other outcome events during the first 6 months of life. In addition, children who did not receive three doses of DTP by 1 year of age or who had incomplete vaccination records were excluded in this analysis. (For the main analysis, they were included.) The final cohort included 103,043 children. Of these children, 2,471 were preterm, and data were not presented on these children because none of them were diagnosed with autism. The final cohort included 100,572 term children.

Exposure to mercury was classified in three categories: those receiving doses of DTP or DT-containing vaccines by 3 months of age (93 days), with a maximum cumulative exposure of 50 μg; by 4 months of age (124 days), with a maximum cumulative exposure of 75 μg; and age-specific exposure by 6 months of age. The researchers examined autism and other neurodevelopmental outcomes that were also examined in the VSD study (Verstraeten et al., 2003). Autism diagnoses in the GPRD were converted from Read and OXMIS codes (coding used by GPRD) to ICD codes. Validation of autism diagnosis was not conducted, but other studies using GPRD data have demonstrated a high degree of reliability in the autism diagnosis (Black et al., 2002; Kaye et al., 2001). A Cox proportional hazards survival was the method of analysis. Survival began at 183 days of age to age of event, censoring occurred at age of event or last date of follow-up, and the results were reported as a hazard ratio per DTP or DT dose.

Overall, there were 104 reports of autism. Cases had a median age at first recorded diagnosis of autism of 4.4 years, at least 8 years of follow-up, and 89 percent of all cases occurred in males. The hazard ratio for autism after receiving doses by 3 months was 0.89 (95% CI, 0.65-1.21; $p = 0.46$); after receiving doses by 4 months was 0.94 (0.73-1.21; $p = 0.66$); and after receiving all doses by 6 months of age was 0.99 (0.88-1.12; $p = 0.89$). Estimates were adjusted for sex and year of birth. The results do not suggest that exposure to thimerosal at these doses increases the risk of autism. A reverse Kaplan-Meier plot was used to illustrate that the results did not suggest an increased risk of autism, and it was used to compare the risk of autism at zero, one, two, and three doses of receiving the DTP vaccine. Miller concluded that there was no evidence that increased exposure to thimerosal at a young age increases the risk of autism.

Unpublished Ecological Study

United States. An unpublished ecological analysis comparing aggregate trends in autism rates in California with the trends in mercury exposure from TCVs was presented to the committee (Blaxill, 2001). To estimate the average level of mercury exposure for children 19-35 months of age in a given year, the mercury content of all recommended vaccine doses (assumed to be 37.5 µg for three doses of hepatitis B, 75 µg for three doses of Hib, and 75-100 µg for three or four doses of DTP) was weighted by estimates from the National Health Interview Survey of coverage rates for the specific vaccines for the specified year. Estimates of the number of children with autism were obtained from annual caseload data from the California Department of Developmental Services database. The presenter concluded that the increasing trends seen in these data, both in the prevalence of autism and the levels of mercury exposure from TCVs, are consistent with the hypothesis that mercury exposure had a direct role in an increasing incidence of autism in the 1990s.

As noted in previous IOM reports (IOM, 1994a,b, 2001b), a positive ecological correlation constitutes only weak evidence of causality, and additional research would be needed to establish a causal association. The analytical value of the California data is limited by the inability to account for any changes over time in diagnostic concepts, case definitions, or age of diagnosis (Fombonne, 2001a). As a result, the committee cannot assess trends in the prevalence of autism from these data. The committee concludes that this unpublished ecological analysis is uninformative with respect to causality.

Several studies show that the prevalence of autism has increased in the past 20 to 30 years, but it is unclear whether the increase derives from changes in case definition, changes in case-finding methods, simply an increased awareness of autism, or other causes (Croen et al., 2002; Fombonne, 1999, 2002, 2003; Gillberg and Wing, 1999; Gurney et al., 2003; Wing and Potter, 2002). Incidence rates are more sensitive measures than prevalence rates for determining changes in the factors causing autism, but only a few incidence studies have been conducted, and the methods used in these studies limit their ability to test this hypothesis (Fombonne, 2003; Wing and Potter, 2002). Further study and clarification about the epidemiology of autism, especially studies examining autism incidence, would be helpful in elucidating why autism has been increasing in the past 30 years.

Causality Argument

Epidemiological studies examining TCVs and autism, including three controlled observational studies (Hviid et al., 2003; Miller, 2004; Verstraeten et al., 2003) and two uncontrolled observational studies (Madsen et al., 2003; Stehr-Green et al., 2003), consistently provided evidence of no association between TCVs and autism, despite the fact that these studies utilized different methods and examined different populations (in Sweden, Denmark, the United States, and the United Kingdom) (see Table 9). Other studies reported findings of an association. These include two ecological studies (Geier and Geier, 2003a, 2004a), three studies using passive reporting data (Geier and Geier, 2003a,b,d), one unpublished study using VSD data (Geier and Geier, unpublished), and one unpublished uncontrolled study (Blaxill, 2001). However, the studies by Geier and Geier cited above have serious methodological flaws and their analytic methods were nontransparent making their results uninterpretable, and therefore noncontributory with respect to causality (see preceding text for discussion). The study by Blaxill is uninformative with respect to causality because of its methodological limitations. Thus, based on this body of evidence, **the committee concludes that the evidence favors rejection of a causal relationship between thimerosal-containing vaccines and autism.**

This conclusion differs from the committee's finding in its 2001 report on TCVs and NDDs which was that the evidence was "inadequate to accept or reject a causal relationship between exposure to thimerosal from childhood vaccines and the neurodevelopmental disorders of autism, ADHD, and speech and language delay." (IOM, 2001b, p. 66) The committee's conclusion in 2001 was based on the fact that there were no published epidemiological studies examining the potential association between TCVs and NDDs, and the two unpublished, epidemiological studies that were available (Blaxill, 2001; Verstraeten, 2001) provided only weak and inconclusive evidence of an association between TCVs and NDDs. Furthermore, the conclusion in the 2001 report pertained to a broader set of NDDs, while this report's conclusion applies *only* to autism.

MMR and Autism

In 1998, Wakefield and colleagues published a case series describing 12 children with pervasive developmental disorder characterized by GI symptoms

TABLE 9 Evidence Table: Exposure to Thimerosal-containing Vaccines and Autism

Citation	Design	Population	Assessment of Vaccine Exposure
Hviid et al. (2003)	Cohort	467,450 children born in Denmark between 1/1/1990 and 12/31/1996.	Whole-cell pertussis doses administered before 6/1/92 were considered to contain thimerosal. Doses administered afterward were considered thimerosal free. Date of vaccination obtained from the National Board of Health. Whole-cell pertussis vaccine administered at 5 weeks, 9 weeks, and 10 months. Thimerosal content was 50 μg (~25 μg of EtHg) in the first dose and 100 μg (~50 μg of EtHg) in each succeeding dose.

Outcomes	Results	Comment	Contribution to Causality Argument
Autism (ICD-10 code F84.0) Autistic spectrum disorders (ICD-10 codes F84.1-F84.9) obtained from the Danish Psychiatric Central Register. Child psychiatrists diagnose and assign diagnostic codes for this register.	*Rate ratio (95% CI) in children vaccinated with at least one dose of wP w/ thimerosal to children vaccinated with a thimerosal-free wP* Adjusted for age and calendar period: Autism 0.85 (0.60-1.20) Other autistic spectrum disorders 1.12 (0.88-1.43) RRs were similar when adjusted for age, calendar period, sex, birthplace, birthweight, 5-minute Apgar score, gestational age, mother's age at birth of child, mother's country of birth *Rate ratio (95%CI) of autism or autistic spectrum disorders of those who received one or more doses of TCVs* Autism one dose: 0.99 (0.59-1.68)* 1.01 (0.60-1.71)** two doses 0.71 (0.46-1.09)* 0.70 (0.46-1.09)** three doses 0.96 (0.63-1.46)* 0.96 (0.63-1.47)** Trend increase in RR per 25 μg et Hg 0.98 (0.90-1.06)* 0.98 (0.90-1.06)**	Authors reanalyzed their results to assess the possibility of misclassification bias, robustness of the results, and the effect of missing values. For assessing misclassification bias, subjects who were vaccinated from 6/1/92 through 12/31/92 were excluded. To evaluate robustness of results, cohort was limited to include only children born between 1991 and 1993. To evaluate the impact of missing values, single imputation was used to replace a missing value with the most common value of the relevant variable. Findings were similar to original analysis. The committee considered the study as having strong internal validity with the findings demonstrating a secular trend increase in autism, even after the removal of	The study shows no association between TCVs and autism.

continued

TABLE 9 Continued

Citation	Design	Population	Assessment of Vaccine Exposure
Verstraeten et al. (2003)	Retrospective cohort Phase 1	Children born from 1/92 to 12/98 at HMO A and B. HMO A: 13,337 HMO B: 110,833	Vaccine history obtained from computerized databases in the HMO. Exposure to thimerosal was based on the mean mercury content of each vaccine in multidose vials. Cumulative exposure at 1, 3, and 7 months of life.

Outcomes	Results	Comment	Contribution to Causality Argument
	Other ASDs one dose: 0.96 (0.67-1.39)* 0.95 (0.66-1.37)** two doses 1.20 (0.92-1.56)* 1.20 (0.92-1.56)** three doses 1.11 (0.83-1.48)* 1.13 (0.84-1.51)** Trend (increase in RR per 25 μg in et Hg) 1.03 *Adjusted for calendar period and age ** Adjusted for age, calendar period, child's sex, child's birthplace, birth weight, 5-minute Apgar score, gestational age, mother's age at birth of child, mother's country of birth	thimerosal in the vaccines used in Denmark. The committee identified a few limitations, including the time-series design of the study and the generalizability of the study's findings to the U.S. situation, especially in regard to the different dosing schedule used in Denmark, and the genetic homogeneity of the Danish population.	
ICD-9-CM (299.0) of autism diagnosis codes in VSD database. Other outcomes included other childhood psychosis, stammering, tics, sleep disorders, eating disorders, emotional disturbances, ADD, developmental language delay, developmental speech delay, coordination disorder.	HMO A: Autism cases : 21 children No RR calculated HMO B: Autism cases: 202 children *RR by increase of 12.5 μg of Hg exposure from TCV (95% CI):* 1 month cum Hg: 1.16 (0.78-1.71) 3 month cum Hg: 1.06 (0.88-1.28) 7-month cum Hg: 1.00 (0.90-1.09) *RR of autism of cum Hg exposure (95% CI) at 3 months*	Validity of autism diagnosis: HMO A: 92.3% HMO B: 81.3% Autism was not analyzed in Phase II because no associations were found between TCV and autism in Phase I.	The study shows no association between TCVs and autism.

continued

TABLE 9 Continued

Citation	Design	Population	Assessment of Vaccine Exposure
Madsen et al. (2003)	Ecological	Denmark children (aged 2-10 years) diagnosed with autism between January 1, 1971 and December 31, 2000.	Thimerosal in vaccines between 1961 to March 1992. 1961-1970: In DTP vaccines given in 4 doses at 5, 6, 7, and 15 months of age. 1970-1992: wP given in three doses when child was 5 and 9 weeks, and at 10 month of age.

Outcomes	Results	Comment	Contribution to Causality Argument
	0-25 µg Hg: 1.00 37.5-50 µg Hg: 1.61 (0.77-3.34) ≥ 62.5 µg Hg: 1.38 (0.55-3.48) chi-square: 1.84 p-value: .40		
	RR of autism of cum Hg exposure (95% CI) at 7 months 0-75 µg Hg: 1.00 87-162.5 µg Hg: 0.96 (0.62-1.46) ≥ 175: 0.65 (0.27-1.52) chi-square: 1.08 p-value: 0.58		
	Relative risks were calculated for those outcomes that contained 50 or more children.		
Psychosis proto-infantilis (ICD-8 299.00); psychosis infantalis posterior (ICD-8 299.01); or since 1994, infantile autism (ICD-10: F84.0) or atypical autism (ICD-10 F84.1) From Danish Psychiatric Central Research Register Only psychiatric inpatient treatment reported between 1969 and 1995.	*Trend data* Incidence rates were calculated for each year between 1971 and 2000. Age and gender specific numbers of people in Denmark were used as a denominator. Autism began to increase in 1991, but continued to increase after discontinuation of thimerosal.	The authors found no increase in incidence of autism during the period when thimerosal was used up to 1990. The authors stated that autism incidence after 1995 may have been exaggerated due to the change in including outpatient cases into the Danish Psychiatric Central Register. Another possible limitation is its generalizability to the U.S. situation.	The study shows no association between TCVs and autism. The study design limits the study's contribution to the causality argument.

continued

TABLE 9 Continued

Citation	Design	Population	Assessment of Vaccine Exposure
Stehr-Green et al. (2003)	Ecological	Children born in Sweden from 1980 to 1996.	Data were collected on vaccination coverage since 1980. Amount of thimerosal in vaccines used in Sweden and time period of its use were obtained from the Swedish Institute for Infectious Disease Control. The average cumulative dose of ethylmercury from vaccine for each birth cohort was calculated by multiplying the amount of ethylmercury in TCV used in Sweden by the vaccine-specific coverage level for Swedish children aged <2 years.
Stehr-Green et al. (2003)	Ecological	Children with neurological disorders who had been admitted to a psychiatric hospital or received outpatient care prior to 1994. The number of autism cases diagnosed among 2- to 10-year-olds was totaled for each year between 1983 and 2000.	Data collected on vaccination coverage levels in Denmark since 1981. Data provided in the Danish Statens Serum Institut include the amount of thimerosal in vaccines used in Denmark and the associated time period. Between 1970 and 1989,

Outcomes	Results	Comment	Contribution to Causality Argument
Outpatient activities reported 1995 and afterward.			
All cases of autism diagnosed in inpatient settings among 2- to 10- year-olds between 1987 to 1999. Outcomes included infantile autism, including atypical autism: ICD-9 codes 299.x for 1987-1997 and ICD-10 codes F84.x for 1997-1999.	*Autism incidence among Swedish inpatients ages 2-10 years old:* Before 1985: 5-7 inpatient-diagnosed cases/100,000 person-years 1993: 9.2 cases/100,000 Thimerosal In DTP until 1979; in DT until 1992. Both had a concentration of 0.01% of thimerosal. Small number of children received thimerosal-containing single-antigen Hib vaccine or acellular pertussis used in a clinical trial prior to 1992. Very small number of children born to high-risk mothers (<1% of annual birth cohort) who may have received thimerosal-containing hep B vaccine.	The authors concluded that the study did not demonstrate a correlation between thimerosal in vaccines and autism rates because autism rates continued to increase after the elimination of thimerosal from vaccines used in Sweden. The authors discuss possible limitations, including the fact that the data from Sweden only reflected cases diagnosed in inpatient settings. The autism increase may result from changes in diagnostic criteria and increasing awareness of autism and related disorders.	The study shows no association between TCVs and autism. The study design limits the study's contribution to the causality argument.
Psychosis proto-infantalis (ICD-8 299.00) Psychosis infantilis posterior (ICD-8 299.01) From 1994 onward Infantile autism (ICD-10 F85)	*Number of cases* Before 1990: <10 cases among 2- to 10- year-olds 1999: 181 cases *Estimated prevalence in 2000*: 8.1 cases/10,000 persons.	The authors concluded that the results did not support the hypothesis that TCVs are responsible for increasing autism rates. Possible reasons for the	

continued

TABLE 9 Continued

Citation	Design	Population	Assessment of Vaccine Exposure
			thimerosal used only in whole-cell pertussis containing vaccines at a concentration of 0.01%. Children in Denmark who received three recommended doses of thimerosal containing wP between 1970 and 1991 would have received 125 μg cum EtHg by age 10 months. Thimerosal entirely eliminated by end of 1992.
Geier and Geier (2003b)	Study design is indeterminate. Classified as ecological because it relies on aggregate data for its analyses.	*Received thimerosal containing vaccine:* DTaP vaccinees who received the vaccine between 1992 through 2000. *Received thimerosal-free vaccine:* DTaP vaccinees who received the vaccine between 1997 and 2000.	TCVs administered from 1992 through 2000; thimerosal-free vaccines administered between 1997 and 2000. Data from the BSS of the CDC were used to calculate the "incidence rates" of autism after vaccination.
Geier and Geier (2003a)	Passive reporting system	Cases: VAERS reports of autism, personality disorders, and mental retardation. Controls: the number of febrile seizures, fevers, pain, edema, and vomiting following vaccine administration.	Thimerosal-containing DTaP vaccine: administered between 1997 and 2001. Thimerosal-free DTaP vaccine administered between 1997 and 2001. Comparison of DTaP vaccine. Thimerosal content based on manufacturers.

Outcomes	Results	Comment	Contribution to Causality Argument
Atypical autism (ICD-10 F84.1)		autism increase may result from changes in the inclusion criteria in the national register and diagnostic changes (from ICD-8 diagnostic coding to ICD-10). Also, prior to 1992, cases did not include those diagnosed in one large clinic. Another possible limitation is its generalizability to the U.S. situation.	
Based on VAERS data. Autism as stated in the descriptions of those reporting autism and in defined fields in the VAERS database.	*Relative Risk of Autism:* 6.0 (P < 0.05) *Attributable Risk:*[1] 5.0 (P < 0.002) *Percent Association:*[2] 86 (P < 0.05) See text for more details.	These studies, which claim to show a link between TCVs and autism, have serious methodological flaws. Please see text for more details.	The results are uninterpretable, and therefore noncontributory, with respect to causality
Autism, personality disorders, and mental retardation as reported in VAERS reports or as defined by fields in the VAERS database. "Incidence"[3] of adverse event was the frequency of the adverse event, as reported in VAERS,	*Odds Ratios* **Autism:** 2.6; OR increased by 0.029 per µg of mercury **Personality disorders:** 1.5; OR increased by 0.012 per µg of mercury **Mental retardation:** 2.5; OR increased by 0.048 µg of mercury	This study, which claims to show a link between TCVs and autism, has serious methodological flaws. Please see text for more details.	The results are uninterpretable, and therefore noncontributory, with respect to causality

continued

TABLE 9 Continued

Citation	Design	Population	Assessment of Vaccine Exposure
			The number of doses "administered" by each manufacturer was determined by data from the BSS.
			The number of adverse events were categorized into two groups: one group receiving an average of 37.5 µg of Hg and the other receiving an average of 87.5 µg of Hg.
Geier and Geier (2003a)	Study design is indeterminate. Classified as ecological because it relies on aggregate data for its analyses.	Birth cohorts from 1984, 1985, 1990-1994 1984 was established as the baseline year.	Amount of mercury received via immunizations (averaged for each birth cohort) as reported in the BSS.
Geier and Geier (2003d)	a) Passive reporting system	Cases: VAERS reporting autism, speech disorders, and heart arrest. "Controls": the number of febrile seizures, fevers, pain, edema, and vomiting following each vaccine.	Thimerosal-containing DTaP vaccine: administered between 1997 and 2001. Thimerosal-free DTaP vaccine administered between 1992 and 2000. Comparison of DTaP

Outcomes	Results	Comment	Contribution to Causality Argument
divided by the number of vaccines administered, according to the BSS.	Data not shown for febrile seizure, fever, pain, edema, and vomiting. Incidence rates not available. See text for more details.		
Autism, speech disorders, orthopedic impairments, visual impairments, deaf-blindness as reported in the 2001 U.S. DOE report.	*Odds ratio* **Autism:** 2.5; OR increased by 0.014 μg of mercury **Speech disorders:** 1.4; OR increased by 0.12 μg of mercury ORs were significantly higher than 1984 baseline measurement. Authors note that there is a linear relationship between increasing mercury from thimerosal in childhood vaccines and odds ratio for NDD.	This study, which claims to show a link between TCVs and autism, has serious methodological flaws. Please see text for more details.	The results are uninterpretable, and therefore noncontributory, with respect to causality
NDDs reported in VAERS, specifically autism, speech disorders, and heart arrest. "Control" adverse events include febrile seizures,	No estimates of relative risk reported. Authors plot "relative risk" to mercury dose. Graphical depiction of the relative risks (DTaP TCV vs. DTaP thimerosal-free vaccines and DTwP TCV vs. DTaP thimerosal-free	This study, which claims to show a link between TCVs and autism, has serious methodological flaws. Please see text for more details.	The results are uninterpretable, and therefore noncontributory, with respect to causality

continued

TABLE 9 Continued

Citation	Design	Population	Assessment of Vaccine Exposure
			vaccine administered from 1997 to 2000. Thimerosal content based on manufacturers.
			The number of doses administered by each manufacturer was determined by data from the BSS.
			The number of adverse events were categorized into two groups: one group receiving an average of 37.5 µg of Hg and the other receiving an average of 87.5 µg of Hg.
Geier and Geier (2003d)	b) Study design is indeterminate. Classified as ecological because it relies on aggregate data for its analyses.	Birth cohorts from 1984, 1985, 1990, 1991, 1992, 1993, 1994	Amount of mercury received via immunizations (averaged for each birth cohort) as reported in the BSS.

Outcomes	Results	Comment	Contribution to Causality Argument
fevers, pain, edema, and vomiting.	vaccine) for autism, speech disorders, and heart arrest versus mercury dose demonstrated increasing trends. In contrast, the authors note that the increased relative risks for febrile seizure, fever, pain, edema, and vomiting did not correlate with an increasing amount of mercury.		
Prevalence of autism, speech disorders, orthopedic impairments, visual impairments, deaf-blindness as reported in the 2001 U.S. DOE report	No estimates of relative risk reported. Authors plot the "prevalence" of autism per 100,000 children versus the amount of mercury dose received per child. The graphs depict an increasing trend between prevalence and amount of mercury dose. As a comparison, the authors plot the prevalence of visual impairments, deaf-blindness, and orthopedic impairments to the amount of mercury dose received by each child. The authors note that these conditions were not associated with the increasing amount of mercury received by each child.	This study, which claims to show a link between TCVs and autism, has serious methodological flaws. Please see text for more details.	The results are uninterpretable, and therefore noncontributory, with respect to causality

continued

TABLE 9 Continued

Citation	Design	Population	Assessment of Vaccine Exposure
Geier and Geier (2004a)	Study design is indeterminate. Classified as ecological because it relies on aggregate data for its analyses.	Birth cohorts 1981, 1982, 1983, 1984, 1985, 1990, 1991, 1992, 1993, 1994, 1995, 1996	Vaccine exposure for each birth cohort was based on the number of vaccines distributed according to CDC's BSS; thimerosal content in each vaccine was based on information from the IOM 2001 report. Vaccines included DTwP, DTaP, DTwP-Hib, DTaP-Hib, Hib, and pediatric HepB.
Geier and Geier (2004b) Unpublished	Data from VSD	Received thimerosal-free DTaP vaccine: 28,056 Received thimerosal-containing DTaP vaccine: 55,335	Vaccine exposure based on receipt of four doses of DTaP vaccine.
Miller (2004) In press	Cohort	Children born 1988-1992 into GPRD practice.	Vaccine information was obtained from GPRD database.
Blaxill (2001; Unpublished)	Ecological	California births from 1985 to 1998.	Average level of mercury for children 19-35 months of age per year. Mercury content of all recommended vaccine doses was weighted by estimates from the National Health Interview Survey of coverage rates for the specific vaccines for the specified year.

Outcomes	Results	Comment	Contribution to Causality Argument
Autism as reported in the DOE report	The prevalence of autism per 100,000 children was plotted against the average mercury dose per child (micrograms). The linear plot demonstrated a slope of 1.6 and the linear regression coefficient was 0.94.[4] The autism OR compared to the increased average mercury dose was plotted; however, no ORs were reported. The slope of the line was 0.023, and the linear regression coefficient was 0.89.	This study, which claims to show a link between TCVs and autism, has serious methodological flaws. Please see text for more details.	The results are uninterpretable, and therefore noncontributory, with respect to causality
ICD-9 299.0 diagnostic code, as reported in VSD database.	*Relative risk for autism:* 9.6 *Attributable risk:* 3.04 per 10,000 children; $p < 0.005$	This study, which claims to show a link between TCVs and autism, has serious methodological flaws. Please see text for more details.	The results are uninterpretable, and therefore noncontributory, with respect to causality
Autism diagnoses in the GPRD were converted from Read and OXMIS codes to ICD codes.	*Hazard ratio (95% CI)* Doses by 3 months: 0.89 (0.65-1.21, $p = 0.40$) Doses by 4 months: 0.94 (0.72-1.21; $p = 0.66$) All doses by 6 months: 0.99 (0.88-1.12; $p = 0.89$)	The author concluded that there was no evidence that increased exposure to thimerosal at a young age increases the risk of autism.	The study shows no association between TCVs and autism.
Estimates of the number of children with autism were obtained from the annual caseload data of the California Department of Developmental Services database.	Increasing trends both in the prevalence of autism and the levels of mercury exposure from TCVs.	The analytical value of the California data is limited by the inability to account for any changes over time in diagnostic concepts, case definitions, or age of diagnosis	The study is uninformative with respect to causality based on the methodological limitations.

continued

TABLE 9 Continued

Citation	Design	Population	Assessment of Vaccine Exposure

[1]The authors used the epidemiologic measure "attributable risk" incorrectly. As noted by Mann (2003), attributable risk is intended to be a measure of the absolute, rather than the relative, difference in risk among the exposed and unexposed groups. Attributable risk percent, known also as the attributable fraction for the exposed or the etiologic fraction, is defined as (risk among the exposed − risk among the unexposed)/(risk among the exposed) and is mathematically equivalent to (RR−1)/RR × 100. Attributable risk percent is interpreted as the proportion of exposed cases whose disease can be attributed to exposure. A second related concept is the population attributable risk percent (also known as attributable fraction for the population) and is defined as (risk in the population − risk for the unexposed)/(risk in the population). Mathematically equivalent formulas are: (prevalence of exposure among cases) × (RR−1)/RR and (prevalence of exposure in the population) × (RR−1)/(1 + prevalence of exposure in the population) × (RR−1). Geier and Geier (2003b) calculate attributable risk by subtracting 1 from the relative risk value (RR−1= attributable risk). Making attributable risk a

and developmental regression (Wakefield et al., 1998). In eight of the cases, parents or physicians reported the onset of these symptoms within 2 weeks of the child's MMR vaccination. This study put forth a hypothesis that a new variant of autism characterized by GI symptoms and developmental regression could be associated with the MMR vaccine. Ten of the original 13 authors have since formally retracted that interpretation: "We wish to make it clear that in this paper no causal link was established between MMR vaccine and autism, as the data were insufficient. However, the possibility of such a link was raised and consequent events have had major implications for public health. In view of this, we consider now is the appropriate time that we should together formally retract the interpretation placed upon these findings in the paper, according to precedent" (Murch et al., 2004).

In response to public concern about the safety of the MMR vaccine following the 1998 study, researchers initiated a number of epidemiological studies to

Outcomes	Results	Comment	Contribution to Causality Argument
		(Fombonne, 2001a). As a result, the committee cannot assess trends in the prevalence of autism from these data. The committee concludes that this unpublished ecological analysis is uninformative with respect to causality.	

fraction of the relative risk provides no information on the absolute or actual risk of thimerosal, nor does it provide information on the proportions of disease either among the exposed or population that can be attributed to exposure.

[2]Percent association, which the authors define as [RR/{RR+1} × 100], is not a recognized epidemiologic measure.

[3]The epidemiologic measure "incidence rate" is used incorrectly in this study. VAERS cannot be used to calculate incidence rates because VAERS does not have complete reporting of all adverse events and because many reports lack a confirmed diagnosis or a confirmed attribution to a vaccine.

[4]The authors appear to use the term "linear regression coefficient" in their analyses to refer to the coefficient of determination (R-sq), although these are distinct concepts. Slope (or partial slope) and coefficient are generally interchangeable terms in the context of regression. Data and variables used in these regression models were not included.

examine the association between the vaccine and ASD. In addition to case reports from VAERS and other sources, the committee identified 16 epidemiological studies related to MMR and autism that were published since the original Wakefield paper. Ten of these studies (DeStefano et al., 2004; DeWilde et al., 2001; Farrington et al., 2001; Fombonne and Chakrabarti, 2001; Geier and Geier, 2003c, 2004a; Madsen et al., 2002; Makela et al., 2002; Takahashi et al., 2003; Taylor et al., 2002) were published since the committee's last review in 2001. These studies addressed four main questions: (1) Are rates of ASD higher among children who are vaccinated with MMR than in those who are not? (2) Is there an increase in ASD as a result of the MMR vaccine? (3) Is there a new variant form of autism associated with the MMR vaccine? and (4) Is the development of ASD temporally associated with receipt of the MMR vaccine? (Wilson et al., 2003).

The studies were conducted in five different countries (the United States, the United Kingdom, Finland, Denmark, and Sweden), using 11 distinct data sources (one data source was used three times and another was used twice). The studies employed a variety of study designs, including time-series analysis, cross-sectional analysis, ecologic analysis, case control, and retrospective cohort. They also differed in how ASD was diagnosed, though most of them relied on service records of children with autism or children with disabilities or on ICD codes (Wilson et al., 2003). All the epidemiological studies of MMR and autism, including those reviewed in the previous IOM report (IOM, 2001a), are described in detail below and are summarized in Table 10.

Controlled Observational Studies

United States. DeStefano and colleagues (2004) conducted a case-control study in the metropolitan Atlanta area comparing ages at first MMR vaccination of a population-based sample of children with autism and school-matched controls who did not have autism. The authors stated that implicit in the exposure comparison was the assumption that if MMR vaccination increases the risk of autism (typical onset is 24 months), children who receive the vaccine at earlier ages would have a higher risk of developing autism. The researchers chose this study design because they did not have full information on onset of initial parental concern, date of first diagnosis of autism, or onset of regression.

Children with autism who were enrolled in the study were identified from the Metropolitan Atlanta Developmental Disabilities Surveillance Program (MADDSP), a population-based surveillance program that monitors the occurrence of selected developmental disabilities among children in the Atlanta region. Autism cases were identified through screening and abstraction of files at multiple sources, including schools, hospitals, clinics, and specialty providers. In 1996, the first year that autism was included as part of the MADDSP, 987 children 3-10 years old with autism were identified. School immunization records were located for 660 of those children; the rest either moved out of the state or transferred to a school outside the Atlanta public school system. Three control children were matched for 97 percent of the children with autism. Controls were selected from the regular education programs and were matched on the basis of age, gender, and school. Data on immunization history was abstracted from immunization forms required for school entry. Case and control children with missing or incomplete vaccination forms[22] were excluded. After all exclusions, 624 cases and 1,824 controls remained in the study.

A developmental pediatrician reviewed the MADDSP data files and classified children with autism into three subgroups with potentially different environmental susceptibilities to development of autism. These non-mutually exclusive groups included (1) children with no indication of developmental delay before

---

[22]Incomplete forms included those that did not list DPT by age 2 or who never listed MMR.

1 year of age (i.e., before recommended age of the first MMR vaccine) or a preexisting condition (e.g., major birth defect, co-occurring developmental disability, or major perinatal or postnatal insult that could have contributed to developmental delays); (2) children with loss of age-appropriate developmental skills (regression) or appropriate skills that failed to progress (plateau); (3) children with and without coexisting mental retardation (defined as an IQ of less than 70).

In addition to vaccination records for all children, researchers obtained additional developmental disability-related information from MADDSP, including birth defects, epilepsy, IQ level, and presence of other developmental disabilities, for children with autism. Demographic data were collected for all case and control children. Approximately 56 percent of cases and controls were matched with Georgia state birth records, which provided additional information about birth and maternal factors (e.g., birth weight and gestational age, and mother's parity, age, race, and education).

The overall distribution of ages at MMR vaccination was similar to that of matched control children; 70.5 percent of cases and 67.5 percent of control children were vaccinated between 12 and 17 months of age. The authors analyzed associations between MMR vaccine and autism using three age cutoffs: (1) < 18 months, as an indicator of on-time vaccination; (2) < 24 months of age, the age at which developmental problems have become apparent in most children with autism; and (3) < 36 months of age, the age by which characteristics of autism must have developed in order to meet DSM-IV criteria. Similar proportions of children received the MMR vaccine by the recommended age of 18 months and before 24 months, the age at which developmental delays are normally recognized in children with autism.

Conditional logistic regression models were used to estimate adjusted ORs. The rates of vaccination prior to 36 months were higher among cases (93.4 percent) than among controls (90.6 percent) (OR = 1.49; 95% CI 1.04-2.14 in the total sample; OR = 1.23; 95% CI 0.64-2.36 in the birth certificate sample).[23] This association was strongest in the age group of 3- to 5-year-olds. The authors suggested that this likely reflected immunization requirements for early intervention programs.

The authors identified several strengths of the study. It was a large population-based study with a well-defined case and control population. In addition, a panel of autism experts reviewed case records to confirm that cases met the DSM-IV criteria. Immunization records were obtained from standardized school records, thus eliminating possibility of recall bias. Data on clinical and behavioral factors and vaccination data were obtained from independent sources, thereby

---

[23]The birth certificate sample was analyzed using a conditional logistic regression model stratified by matching variables (age, gender, and school), and was adjusted for birth weight, multiple gestation, maternal age, and maternal education (DeStefano et al., 2004).

TABLE 10 Evidence Table: Exposure to MMR Vaccine and Autism

Citation	Design	Population	Assessment of Vaccine Exposure
DeStefano et al. (2004)	Case-control (Controlled observational)	624 cases and 1,824 controls who were ages 3-10 years old in 1996 *Cases:* Population-based sample of children with autism in Atlanta metro area *Controls:* Children selected from regular education programs in Atlanta metro area and matched on age (in 1996), gender, and school	Immunization history abstracted from immunization forms required for school entry. Demographic data collected for all children.

Outcomes	Results	Comment	Contribution to Causality Argument
Autistic cases identified through MADDSP, a population-based surveillance program monitoring the occurrence of select disabilities among children in the Atlanta metro area. Additional disability-related information, including birth defects, epilepsy, IQ level, and other disabilities collected from MADDSP. Additional data on birth and maternal characteristics was collected on a subset of children who had Georgia birth certificates.	Conditional logistic regression model stratified by matched control sets was used to estimate odds ratios. Associations with autism analyzed using three specific vaccination age cutoffs (1) <18 months; (2) <24 months; (3) <36 months. A subanalysis was conducted of children with Georgia birth certificates to evaluate potential confounders in terms of birth and maternal characteristics. Similar proportions of children received the MMR vaccine by the recommended age of 18 months and <24 months. The rates of vaccination prior to 36 months were higher among cases (93.4%) than among controls (90.6%) (OR=1.49; 95% CI 1.04-2.14 in the total sample); (OR=1.23; 95% CI 0.64-2.36 in birth certificate sample). The association was strongest among the age group of 3- to 5-year-olds.	Similar patterns of age at first MMR vaccination among cases and controls. Similar proportions of cases and controls vaccinated according to ACIP schedule (<18 months) and by typical age of onset of autism (<24 months). Children with autism were more likely to be vaccinated before 26 months of age compared to controls.	The study shows no association between MMR and autism.

continued

TABLE 10 Continued

Citation	Design	Population	Assessment of Vaccine Exposure
Taylor et al. (1999)	Self-matched case series (Controlled observational; Case crossover)	498 children with autism born since 1979 from eight North Thames health districts, UK 261 core autism 166 atypical autism 71 Asperger's syndrome	MMR information was obtained independently from clinical records from the Regional Interactive Child Health Computing System (RICHS)

Outcomes	Results	Comment	Contribution to Causality Argument
Cases with autistic disorders were obtained from special school records and special needs/disability registers at child developmental centers. A pediatric registrar extracted information from clinical records of <16 years of age. Information included age at diagnosis, child's age when parents were first concerned, and age when regression was first noticed. Authors verified autism diagnosis by comparing ICD-10 autism definition to information on the child in clinical records.	*Trends* Core and atypical cases from 1979-1992: Test for zero trend: p < 0.001 Asperger's syndrome from 1979-1992: p = 0.06 Core and atypical autism No evidence of sudden "step up" in 1987 No exponential trend change after MMR vaccine was introduced in 1987 Trends in autism incidence by birth cohort since 1987 were not temporally associated with changes in vaccine coverage. *Difference in age at diagnosis between those vaccinated before or after 18 months of age and those never vaccinated* p = 0.41 *Interaction between vaccine categories and year of birth* p = 0.29 *Fold differences in mean ages (95% CI):* Vaccinated before 18 mos. over unvaccinated: 0.91 (0.79-1.05) Vaccinated after 18 mos. over unvaccinated: 0.93 (0.81-1.08)		The study shows no association between MMR and autism.

continued

TABLE 10 Continued

Citation	Design	Population	Assessment of Vaccine Exposure
Farrington et al. (2001) Updates/ Reanalyzes data from Taylor et al. (2000)	Self-matched case series (also referred to as case crossover) (Controlled observational)	Self-matched case series method (see Taylor et al., 1999, for details), same age groups. Cases: 357	Receipt of MMR vaccine or any measles-containing vaccine (MMR, single-antigen measles, measles and rubella).

Outcomes	Results	Comment	Contribution to Causality Argument
	MMR vaccine *Relative incidence (95% CI)* Autism diagnosis <12 months: 0.94 (0.60-1.47) Autism diagnosis < 24 months: 1.09 (0.79-1.52) Parental concern < 6 months: 1.48 (1.04-2.12) Parental concern < 12 months: 0.90 (0.63-1.29) Regression < 2 months: 0.92 (0.38-2.21) < 4 months: 1.00 (0.52-1.95) <6 months: 0.85 (0.45-1.60)		
Core autism and atypical autism. Autism diagnosis, parental concern, regression.	*Relative incidence (95% CI)* Receipt of MMR vaccine: Autism diagnosis <60: 1.24 (0.67-2.27) Any time after vaccine: 1.06 (0.49-2.30) Parental concern <36: 0.83 (0.50-1.36) Any time after vaccine: 0.76 (0.45-1.27) *Regression* <25: 0.76 (0.33-1.71) Any time after vaccine: 0.66 (0.26-1.66) Receipt of any measles-containing vaccines: Autism diagnosis <60: 0.96 (0.52-1.77) Any time after vaccine: 2.03 (0.80-5.18)	The authors conclude that the results did not support the hypothesis that MMR vaccine or measles-containing vaccine cause autism.	The study shows no association between MMR and autism.

continued

TABLE 10 Continued

Citation	Design	Population	Assessment of Vaccine Exposure
Taylor et al. (2002)	Self-matched case series (also referred to as case crossover) (Controlled observational)	278 children with childhood autism and 195 with atypical autism Children born between 1979 and 1998 in five health districts in east London and identified from computerized disability register	Abstracted information from clinical notes, then linked the information to independent computerized vaccination records in the regional interactive child health system (TotalCare). Researchers also obtained information regarding whether the child received the vaccine before or after parental concern, or whether child had never received the vaccine.

Outcomes	Results	Comment	Contribution to Causality Argument
	Parental concern <36: 0.92 (0.56-1.49) Any time after vaccine: 0.89 (0.54-1.48) Regression <25: 0.76 (0.33-1.71) Any time after vaccine: 0.66 (0.26-1.66)		
Measured bowel problems lasting 3 months Age of reported regression Looking for evidence of a "new variant" form of autism	*Proportion of children with childhood autism and those with atypical autism* Bowel symptoms: w/ childhood autism: 18% w/ atypical autism: 16% p = 0.73 Regression: w/ childhood autism: 23% w/ atypical autism: 27% p = 0.27 *Trends by year of birth (1979-1999) in proportion of children with autism* Bowel symptoms OR: 0.98 (95% CI 0.93-1.04, p = 0.50) Regression OR: 0.98 (95% CI 0.93-1.03, p = 0.47) *Difference between if child receiving the MMR vaccine before or after parental concern* Bowel problems: p = 0.48 Regression: p = 0.83 Regression was reported by parents in 25% of the 469 children cases in which developmental information was recorded.	Authors suggest that the findings provide no support for an MMR associated "new variant" form of autism with developmental regression and bowel problems, and do provide further evidence against involvement of MMR vaccine in the initiation of autism.	The study shows no association between MMR and autism.

continued

TABLE 10 Continued

Citation	Design	Population	Assessment of Vaccine Exposure
Fombonne and Chakrabarti (2001)	Cross-sectional study (Controlled observational)	*Stafford sample*: 96 children born between 1992 and 1995 and diagnosed with pervasive developmental disorder. Autistic disorder = 26 Atypical autism = 56 Asperger syndrome = 13 Childhood disintegrative disorder = 1 Comparison samples: *MHC sample:* 69 children born between 1987 and 1996 with a confirmed diagnosis of PDD. *MFS sample:* 99 subjects born between 1954 and 1979 with an ICD-10 diagnosis of autism.	*Stafford sample:* Community pediatrician who assessed all of the children obtained immunization history from medical data. Immunization dates were verified by comparing information in the Child Health System. 99% of children received the first MMR vaccine; 65.6% received the second MMR *MHC sample:* Authors note that subjects in sample were likely to have been exposed to MMR vaccine based on birth dates. *MFS sample:* None were exposed to the MMR vaccine, based on birth year.

Outcomes	Results	Comment	Contribution to Causality Argument
	Bowel problems reported in children with regression: 26% Without regression: 14% p = 0.002		
Stafford sample: Clinical investigations confirmed PDD diagnosis. Parents were administered the Autism Diagnostic Interview-Revised (ADI-R) by trained registrars to obtain information on symptoms related to regression.	*CDD incidence (95% CI):* 0.6/10,000 (0.02-3.6/10,000) Age at first Parental Concern (standard deviation) Stafford sample: 19.3 (8.7) MHC Sample: 19.2 (8.8) MFS Sample: 19.5 (13.6) $F_{2250} = 0.02$, not significant *Rate of Regressive Autism (standard deviation)*	The authors note several limitations, including small sample size, information about children's GI symptoms were obtained from survey of parents and clinical investigations, and children's guts were not directly examined.	The study shows no association between MMR and autism.
MHC Sample: Subjects were from patients seen at a specialist autism team. *Original study has methods for diagnosis.* Parents were administered the ADI-R by trained registrars to obtain information on symptoms related to regression.	Probable*:* Stafford: 7 (7.3) MFS: 14 (14.3) Definite Stafford: 8 (8.3) MFS 4 (4.1) Any (Probable/Definite) Stafford: 15 (15.6) MFS: 18 (18.4) *Statistical Testing:* Probable and definite: $X^2 = 3.65$; df = 2; p > 0.15		
MFS sample: Data were available for 98 subjects from ADI (first version) and an earlier version of the ADI-R.	Definite only: Fisher's exact test; p = 0.25 Any (Probable/Definite) Fisher's exact test; p = 0.70 *Mean age of children when parents were first concerned*		

continued

TABLE 10 Continued

Citation	Design	Population	Assessment of Vaccine Exposure
DeWilde et al. (2001)	Case control (Controlled observational)	Cases: 71 children with autism Controls: 284 (4 per case) matched for age, sex, month of MMR vaccination, and GP practice	MMR vaccination obtained from records in the Doctor's Independent Network database.

Outcomes	Results	Comment	Contribution to Causality Argument
	(standard deviation) Stafford sample With regression: 19.8 months (7.4)		
	Without regression: 19.3 months (9.0) t = 0.22; df = 94; not significant		
	Mean interval between immunization date and age of children at first parental concern With regression: 248 days Without regression: 272 days t = 0.32; not significant		
	ADI-R scores were not statistically significant between Stafford children with or without regression.		
	No report of inflammatory bowel disorder		
	OR between GI symptoms and regression (95% CI)/ Fisher's exact test: 0.63 (0.06-3.2)/p = 0.86, not significant		
The number of consultations 2 months and 6 months before and after MMR vaccination	*Mean difference in number of consultations 2 months before and after MMR vaccination (95% CI)/ Wilcoxon rank sum test:* -0.05 (-0.54-0.44)/p = 0.45	Authors note that autism diagnosis was not confirmed. Also unclear how receipt of MMR vaccination was validated in subjects. Also unclear when autism was diagnosed.	The study shows no association between MMR and autism.
	Mean difference in number of consultations 6 months before and after MMR vaccination (95% CI)/ Wilcoxon rank sum test: 0.04 (-0.75-0.83)/p = 0.59		

continued

TABLE 10 Continued

Citation	Design	Population	Assessment of Vaccine Exposure
Madsen et al. (2002)	Retrospective cohort (Controlled observational)	Children born in Denmark from January 1991 to December 1998: 537,303 Vaccinated: 440,655 (1,647,504 person-years follow-up) Unvaccinated: 96,648 (482,360 person-years follow-up)	Vaccination information obtained from data reported to the National Board of Health by general practitioners. Information obtained from 1991 to 1999 for MMR vaccination received at 15 months of age.

Outcomes	Results	Comment	Contribution to Causality Argument
	Mean difference in number of consultations before autism diagnosis:		
	60 days before: 1.00 (0.38-1.61)/p = 0.007		
	180 days before: 1.90 (0.81-2.99)/p = 0.009		
Danish Psychiatric Central Register provided information on autism. Diagnoses made in psychiatric hospitals, psychiatric departments, and outpatient clinics in Denmark. Outcomes include autistic disorder (ICD-10 F84.0 and DSM-IV 299.00) and another autistic spectrum disorder (ICD-10 F84.1 through F84.9 and DSM-IV 299.10 and 299.80).	*Adjusted Relative risk of vaccinated vs. unvaccinated children* Autistic disorder: 0.92 (0.68-1.24) Other autistic-spectrum disorders 0.83 (0.65-1.07) Adjusted for age, calendar period, sex, birth weight, gestational age, mother's education, and socioeconomic status. No association between development of autistic disorder and age at vaccination (p = 0.23) Interval since vaccination (p = 0.42) Calendar period at time of vaccination (p = 0.06) Adjustment for potential confounders yielded similar risk estimates.	Consultant in child psychiatry with experience in autism validated the diagnoses in 40 children with autistic disorder. 92% of the diagnoses fit the definition used by the CDC in an autism-prevalence study.	The study shows no association between MMR and autism.

continued

TABLE 10 Continued

Citation	Design	Population	Assessment of Vaccine Exposure
Makela et al. (2002)	Retrospective cohort (Controlled observational)	535,544 1- to 7-year-old children vaccinated between November 1982 and June 1986 in Finland.	MMR vaccination began in 1982 of children age 14 to 18 months and 6 years of age. Data from a surveillance study by the National Public Health Institute. Information also included age at vaccination, timing (year and month) of the first MMR vaccination.
Takahashi et al. (2003)	Case control (Controlled observational)	*Cases:* 21 autistic children born between 1988 and 1992. Two cases were diagnosed with Asperger's syndrome; another case has a regressive clinical course. *Controls:* 42 children matched to cases according to sex and birth year. From Tokyo Metropolitan Umegaoka Hospital.	Immunization history, including vaccination date, vaccine type, lot number, and provider's name were obtained from the Maternal Child Health Handbook. From 1989 to 1993, MMR vaccine/monovalent measles vaccine administered at age 12 months; DTP admistered at 2, 4, and 6 months; OPV administered at 3 and 9 months; BCG administered at 3 months. Monovalent mumps and rubella were given to those who did not receive the MMR vaccine.

Outcomes	Results	Comment	Contribution to Causality Argument
ICD-8 Autistic disorders: 290-299 Psychoses; 95.8 Infantile autism; 308.99 Gerendum abnorme infantum ICD-9 Autistic disorders : 299 Psychoses ex origine infantia 2990 Autismus infantilis 2998 Developmental disorder 2999 Developmental disorder From nationwide hospital discharge register Hospitalizations for autism between November 1982 and December 1995	A total of 352 vaccinees were hospitalized for autism, of which 309 were hospitalized after vaccination. Interval between MMR vaccination and hospitalization was between 3 days to 12 years and 5 months. The authors did not detect clustering in the intervals from vaccination to hospitalization. 43 vaccinated after the first hospitalization; 31 hospitalized but were unvaccinated between November 1982 and June 1986.	The authors note several limitations: autism incidence could not be precise; nonhospitalized autism cases were not included; and some vaccinated children may have been classified as unvaccinated.	The study shows no association between MMR and autism.
Medical records of autistic patients included information on age at initial onset of autistic symptoms, age of diagnosis according to ICD-10 code, and family history of ASD. Diagnosis of autism was made based on DSM-IV definition.	*OR (95% CI) of autism to MMR* Monovalent measles: 5.33 (1.03-27.7) Monovalent mumps: 3.33 (0.45-24.6) Monovalent rubella: 3.82 (0.59-24.7) Nonmeasles: immeasurable Nonmumps: 8 (1.33-48.2) Nonrubella: 8.57) (1.30-56.4	The authors interpret the findings to demonstrate that autism risk after receipt of the MMR vaccine is lower than after receipt of monovalent vaccines. However, the authors note that selection bias, vaccination delay in autistic cases, and the small sample size may have affected the results.	The study shows no association between MMR and autism.

continued

TABLE 10 Continued

Citation	Design	Population	Assessment of Vaccine Exposure
Dales et al. (2001)	Ecological	California children born between 1980 and 1994.	MMR immunization levels between 1980 and 1994 were determined by birth year from the California Department of Health Services Annual surveys of statewide random samples and from public and private school kindergarten immunization records. School immunization records were reviewed to determine age at receipt of immunization. Coverage levels were measured as proportions of children at 17 months in each year's survey who received the MMR vaccine and those at 24 months who received the vaccine.
Geier and Geier (2004a)	Study design is indeterminate. Classified as ecological because it relies on aggregate data for its analyses.	Children with autism from U.S. Department of Education data files	Estimates of primary pediatric measles-containing vaccine coverage for birth cohorts 1982, 1984, 1991-1996

Outcomes	Results	Comment	Contribution to Causality Argument
		There was a significant difference in immunization completeness between cases and controls for mumps, rubella, varicella, and encephalitis vaccination. 87.5% response rate for cases. Controls had 58% response rate.	
Autism cases, as reported to the California Department of Developmental Services. Children were born between 1980 and 1994 and had an ICD-9 code of 299. Other PPD outcomes were excluded.	*Relative increase from 1980 to 1994* MMR coverage by age 24 months: 14% (from 72% to 82%) Number of autism cases: 572% (from 176 cases to 1182 cases) Rate of autism cases: 373% 1980: 44/100,000 births 1994: 208/100,000 births	Ecological nature of this study. The authors note several limitations: Unknown how many autism cases were not accounted for in the system; expansion of the system probably affected the enrollment; the proportion of children born outside of California; diagnostic methods and categorization of people.	The study shows no association between MMR and autism. The study design limits its contribution to the causality argument.
Estimated prevalence by creating birth cohorts for 1982, 1984, and 1991-1996 using age at which child was recorded as having autism.	Plotted estimated number of primary pediatric measles-containing vaccines in comparison to prevalence of autism for each birth cohort examined. Reported slope of the line was 4831[1] and linear regression coefficient was	These studies, which report a link between MMR and autism, have serious methodological flaws. Please see text.	The results are uninterpretable, and therefore noncontributory, with respect to causality.

continued

TABLE 10 Continued

Citation	Design	Population	Assessment of Vaccine Exposure
Geier and Geier (2003c)	Study design is indeterminate. Classified as ecological because it relies on aggregate data for its analyses.	VAERS reports of serious neurologic symptoms following primary pediatric MMR immunization from 1994 to 2000 that developed within 30 days. Comparison group: VAERS reports of vaccine recipients who developed serious neurologic symptoms after DTwP vaccine	Estimates of primary pediatric MMR vaccine coverage and DTwP coverage in birth cohorts from 1994 to 2000 from the CDC's BSS.
Kaye et al. (2001)	Ecological	Birth cohorts 1988-1993 of children registered in the GPRD.	Proportion of children registered in the GPRD who received the MMR vaccine for each annual birth cohort. Children received the vaccine within 60 days of birth and had at least 2 years of recorded follow-up.
Gillberg and Heijbel (1998) Reanalysis of Gillberg et al. (1991)	Ecological	55 Swedish children born 1975-1994 and diagnosed with autism 19 Swedish children born 1975-1994 and diagnosed with autistic like condition	MMR exposure was based on birth year. MMR was introduced for all 18-month-old children in Sweden in 1982.

Outcomes	Results	Comment	Contribution to Causality Argument
	0.91^2 (regression model not specified).		
Serious neurologic symptoms, as reported in VAERS: Cerebellar ataxia, autism, mental retardation, and permanent brain damage.	*Risk estimates of autism after MMR vaccination compared to after DTwP vaccination* Relative risk: 5.2 Attributable risk:[3] 4.2 "Percent Association":[4] 84 Statistical significance: p < 0.001 95% CI: 3.0-9.2	These studies, which report a link between MMR and autism, have serious methodological flaws. Please see text.	The results are uninterpretable, and therefore noncontributory, with respect to causality.
114 boys in the GPRD born between 1988 and 1993 and first diagnosed with autism at ages 2-5 years. The 4-year cumulative incidence of autism was calculated for each birth cohort.	*4 year risk of autism (95% CI)* 1988: 8/10,000 (4-14) 1993: 29/10,000 (20-43) p < 0.0001 by score test for trend in odds MMR prevalence ≈97% for each successive birth annual cohort from 1988 to 1993	The authors note that based on the findings, there was no correlation between autism incidence in each birth cohort (1988-1993) and MMR prevalence: as autism increased from 1988 to 1993, MMR coverage levels remained constant. Limitations include the ecological nature of the study, and the lack of confirmation of autism diagnosis.	The study shows no association between MMR and autism. The study design limits its contribution to the causality argument.
Children were diagnosed with autistic disorder based on DSM-III-R definition. The authors note that autistic-like condition is similar to ICD-10 atypical autism.	*Autistic children who did not receive the MMR vaccine (born between 1/1/1975 and 6/30/1980):* 34 (62%) *Autistic children who received the MMR vaccine (born between 7/1/1980 and 12/31/1984):* 21 (34%)	The authors note that if MMR were related to autism, then more than 45% of children born between 7/1/1980 and 12/31/1984 would have developed autism. Similar results were found	The study shows no association between MMR and autism. The study design limits its contribution to the causality argument.

continued

TABLE 10 Continued

Citation	Design	Population	Assessment of Vaccine Exposure
Patja et al. (2000)	Passive surveillance	1.8 million Finnish people who received the MMR vaccine 1982-1996 (3 million doses of MMR vaccine)	Since 1982, the MMR vaccine was administered twice to children—at ages 14-18 months and again at 6 years of age. Other groups include military recruits, health care workers, nursing school students, and 11- to 13-year-old girls who received the vaccine only once. From 1988 to 1993, rubella-seronegative women were vaccinated after delivery.
Peltola et al. (1998)	Passive surveillance	1.8 million Finnish people who received the MMR vaccine 1982-1996 (3 million doses of MMR vaccine)	Since 1982, the MMR vaccine was administered twice to children—at ages 14-18 months and again at 6 years of age. Other groups include military

Outcomes	Results	Comment	Contribution to Causality Argument
	Autistic-like condition in children who did not receive the MMR vaccine (born between 1/1/1975 and 6/30/1980): 13 (68%) *Autistic-like condition in children who received the MMR vaccine (born between 7/1/1980 and 12/31/1984):* 6 (32%)	for children with autistic-like conditions. The authors concluded that the findings did not support a link between MMR and autistic disorder or atypical autism. Ecological nature of the study limits its ability to assess causality.	
Death, likely allergic reactions, neurologic disorders, miscellaneous events. Reports of adverse events were submitted to the central office by health care personnel, public health nurses, general practitioners, and pediatricians in primary care and hospitals. Reports were evaluated and, if needed, the hospital/health care center was contacted for additional information.	No cases of autism were reported. Vaccine associated adverse events 437 173 serious reactions 169 potentially serious 79 hospitalizations	The authors concluded that there was no evidence to support the hypothesis of association between MMR vaccine and ASD or IBD.	The study shows no association between MMR and autism. The study design limits its contribution to the causality argument.
Gastrointestinal symptoms or signs lasting 24 hours or longer after receipt of the MMR vaccine. Information was	*Autistic spectrum disorder* None reported *Gastrointestinal symptoms* 31 children 20 hospitalized		The study shows no association between MMR and autism. The study design limits its contribution to the

continued

TABLE 10 Continued

Citation	Design	Population	Assessment of Vaccine Exposure
			recruits, health care workers, nursing school students, and 11- to 13-year-old girls who received the vaccine only once. From 1988 to 1993, rubella-seronegative women were vaccinated after delivery.
Wakefield et al. (1998)	Case series	12 children with history of pervasive developmental disorder referred to the Royal Free Hospital and School of Medicine in London, England. Children were between 3 and 10 years of age.	Researchers obtained subject's immunization history from child's parent or doctor.

Outcomes	Results	Comment	Contribution to Causality Argument
obtained from hospital or health center records or from public health nurses.	Symptoms included diarrhea, gingivostomatitis, vomiting only, and abdominal pains. Time between symptom onset and MMR vaccination: 20 hours to 15 days		causality argument.
Children underwent gastroenterological, neurological, and developmental assessment and review of developmental records. Ileocolonoscopy and biopsy sampling, MRI, EEG, lumbar puncture were done under sedation. Barium follow-through was conducted when possible. Biochemical, hematological, and immunologic profiles were examined.	*Number of cases with behavioral problems* Autism: 9 Disintegrative psychosis: 1 Postviral or postvaccinial encephalitis: 2 *Number of cases with intestinal abnormalities* All 12 children had intestinal abnormalities *MMR vaccine* In 8 children, onset of behavioral problems was linked to MMR vaccine by parent or physician 6 children had autism 1 postvaccinial encephalitis None of the children had neurological abnormalities on clinical exam. 5 had adverse reaction to MMR vaccine (rash, fever, delirium), 3 cases had convulsions. Average interval between exposure and 1st behavioral symptom: 6.3 days (range 1-14 days)	Authors did not find association between MMR vaccine and syndrome described. They identified a chronic entercocolitis in children that may be related to neuropsychiatric dysfunction. In most cases, onset of symptoms was after MMR vaccination.	This case series is uninformative with respect to causality.

continued

TABLE 10 Continued

Citation	Design	Population	Assessment of Vaccine Exposure

[1]The reported slope of 4831 seems anomalous.

[2]The authors appear to use the term "linear regression coefficient" in their analyses to refer to the coefficient of determination (R-sq), although these are distinct concepts. Slope (or partial slope) and coefficient are generally interchangeable terms in the context of regression. Data and variables used in these regression models were not included.

[3]The authors used the epidemiologic measure "attributable risk" incorrectly. As noted by Mann (2003), attributable risk is intended to be a measure of the absolute, rather than the relative, difference in risk among the exposed and unexposed groups. Attributable risk percent, known also as the attributable fraction for the exposed or the etiologic fraction, is defined as (risk among the exposed − risk among the unexposed)/(risk among the exposed) and is mathematically equivalent to $(RR-1)/RR \times 100$. Attributable risk percent is interpreted as the proportion of exposed cases whose disease can

reducing potential information bias. The study also controlled for confounding demographic and birth factors.

One limitation of the study was the lack of vaccination records for one-third of the 987 case children, owing to transfers to schools outside the Atlanta public school district. In addition, a subanalysis of children with Georgia birth certificates was conducted to evaluate potential confounders in terms of birth and maternal characteristics. The birth certificate sample did have lower ORs, which could represent random fluctuation or potential bias related to being born outside of Georgia.

United Kingdom. In a population-based, self-matched case series study (or case-crossover study) of children in eight health districts of the North East Thames region in the United Kingdom, Taylor and colleagues (1999) investigated trends in the incidence of ASD before and after the introduction of MMR vaccine (in 1988) and tested for postvaccination clustering of diagnoses or other indicators of onset. Children with ASD born since 1979 were identified from computerized specialized-needs/disability registries and from records in special schools. Information was extracted on the age at which the disorder was diagnosed, the recorded age at which parents first became concerned about the child's developmental course, and the age at which regression became obvious (if it occurred). The authors identified 498 children with ASD: 261 with typical (core) autism, 166 with atypical autism, and 71 with Asperger's syndrome. When ICD-10 criteria were applied to available records, these diagnoses were confirmed for 82 percent of core autism cases, 31 percent of atypical autism cases, and 38 percent of Asperger's syndrome cases. While not all cases were verified according to ICD-10 criteria, most were documented as having been assessed by a specialist clinician. All 498 cases were included in the analyses. Data on the vaccination

Outcomes	Results	Comment	Contribution to Causality Argument

be attributed to exposure. A second related concept is the population attributable risk percent (also known as attributable fraction for the population) and is defined as (risk in the population – risk for the unexposed)/(risk in the population). Mathematically equivalent formulas are: (prevalence of exposure among cases) × (RR–1)/RR and (prevalence of exposure in the population) × (RR–1)/(1 + prevalence of exposure in the population) × (RR–1). Geier and Geier (2003b) calculate attributable risk by subtracting 1 from the relative risk value (RR–1 = attributable risk). Making attributable risk a fraction of the relative risk provides no information on the absolute or actual risk of thimerosal, nor does it provide information on the proportions of disease either among the exposed or population that can be attributed to exposure.

[4]Percent association, which the authors define as [RR/{RR+1} × 100], is not a recognized epidemiologic measure.

histories of these children were obtained from a separate regional information system.

Three statistical analyses were undertaken. First, in a time-series analysis, Poisson regression was used to fit an exponential trend to the number of cases diagnosed by age 60 months for children born between 1979 and 1992. Children born later were excluded because a diagnosis might not have been made by the time of the study. The trend showed a significant increase in cases for core and atypical autism but produced no evidence of a sudden "step up" after MMR vaccine was introduced in the United Kingdom.

The second analysis focused on children born after 1987. Among the 389 study subjects in this group, the proportion who had received MMR vaccine by their second birthday (86.4 percent) was reported to be similar to that of the North East Thames region in general. A further analysis was limited to 356 children who were diagnosed with core or atypical autism at age 18 months or later. Of these cases, 233 received the MMR vaccine before this age, 64 never received it, and 59 received the vaccine at 18 months or later. Children with Asperger's syndrome were excluded because of the small numbers involved and their older age at diagnosis. There were no statistically significant differences in mean age at diagnosis between those vaccinated before 18 months of age, those vaccinated afterward, and those never vaccinated. There was no temporal association between changes in the incidence of autism by birth cohort since 1987 and changes in vaccine coverage.

The third analysis focused on the timing of diagnosis, first parental concern, and regression in children who received one or more MMR vaccine doses. With one exception, the authors found no clustering of diagnosis, parental concern, or autistic regression in the periods following vaccination. (The authors investigated periods within 12 or 24 months after vaccination for diagnosis; periods within 6 or 12 months after vaccination for parental concern; and periods within 2, 4, or 6 months following vaccination for regression.) A statistically significant clustering of parental concern was found within 6 months of vaccination (relative incidence 1.48; 95% CI, 1.04-2.12), and this was attributed to a large peak in recorded parental concern at 18 months and a peak in MMR vaccination at 13 months. Because the convergence of parental reports around age 18 months may reflect recall uncertainty and age 13 months corresponds to the recommended vaccination schedule, this association was interpreted by the authors as an artifact related to the difficulty of precisely defining the onset of symptoms. The authors concluded that their analyses did not support a causal association between MMR vaccination and autism or the onset of autistic regression.

In an extended analysis using the same data as Taylor and colleagues (1999), Farrington and colleagues (2001) assessed the temporal association between MMR vaccine and ASD. This analysis used a self-matched case-series method employing the same age groups as the previous study. The Farrington study found no increase in the incidence of diagnosis of autism, regressive autism, or parental concern at 24, 36, or 60 months following vaccination. There was no increased likelihood of ASD, regression, or parental concern when comparing pre- and postvaccination groups.

United Kingdom. Taylor and colleagues (2002) updated their 1999 analysis in five of the eight health districts studied in North East London to examine the association between the MMR vaccine and bowel problems and developmental regression in children. Using computerized health registers of children with disabilities, information from special schools, and psychiatric records, the investigators identified children with autism who were born between 1979 and 1998. Information abstracted from clinical records was then linked to independent vaccination records. The researchers also recorded information on bowel problems (when they exceeded 3 months in duration), onset of parental concern about the child's development, and regression (if there was documented decline in the child's development or parents reported loss of skills).

A total of 473 children with autism (278 with childhood autism and 195 with atypical autism) were enrolled in the study. Of the 473 children, 81 (17 percent) were reported as having bowel problems. Regression was reported by parents in 118 (25 percent) of the 469 children who had developmental records. The proportion with bowel problems and regression was similar among the children with childhood autism and those with atypical autism.

The researchers conducted single and multivariate logistic regression analyses to examine the relationship between exposure to the MMR vaccine and the onset of autism and the presence of bowel problems and regression. Adjustments were made for several potential confounders (sex, year of birth, district, age of parental concern, type of autism), but the adjustments did not significantly affect the results. No significant trends were found by year of birth in the proportion of children with autism with bowel symptoms (OR = 0.98; 95% CI, 0.93-1.04; p = 0.47) or regression (OR = 0.98; 95% CI, 0.93-1.03; p = 0.50) during the 20-year period from 1979 to 1998.

There was no significant difference in the rates of bowel symptoms or regression between three groups: children with autism who received the MMR vaccination prior to onset of concerns about development (where MMR might have caused the autism); those who received MMR vaccination after the onset of parental concerns; and to those who did not receive the MMR. These results found neither evidence of an association of these two symptoms with the MMR vaccine (p = 0.57) nor a change in the proportion with these symptoms by year of birth (OR = 0.98; 95% CI, 0.89-1.07; p = 0.58).

The authors did find an association between bowel problems and developmental regression in the study population. Thirty-one of the 118 children [26 percent] with regression and 49 of the 351 children [14 percent] (p = 0.002) without regressive autism reported bowel symptoms. Single and multivariable logistic regression models, however, showed no association with these factors and MMR vaccine. The authors suggested that the occurrence of the bowel problems and regression together might reflect particular dietary problems, but that the findings do not support the hypothesis of a MMR-induced new variant form of autism with regression and bowel symptoms.

United Kingdom. Fombonne and Chakrabarti (2001) conducted a cross-sectional study to examine whether a new phenotype of autism, characterized by regression and bowel symptoms, is associated with MMR. The authors stated that if this new phenotype of autism exists, then at least one of the following six predictions should be supported by empirical data: (1) childhood disintegrative disorder (CDD)[24] has become more prevalent; (2) the average age at first parental concern for children with autism who received MMR is closer to the average immunization age than in children who did not receive MMR; (3) developmental regression in children with autism has become more common in MMR-vaccinated children; (4) the age of onset for regressive autism clusters around the MMR immunization date and is different from that of children with autism without regression; (5) children with regressive autism have different symptom and severity profiles than those without regressive autism; or (6) regressive autism is associated with GI symptoms and/or inflammatory bowel disorder.

This study used three samples to examine these questions. The primary sample for this study, the Stafford sample, was drawn from a population-based epidemiologic survey of pervasive developmental disorder (synonymous with

---

[24]CDD is a rare pervasive developmental disorder that applies to children who develop normally until age 2 to 3 and then present with behavioral disintegration and develop severe autism and intellectual impairments (Fombonne and Chakrabarti, 2001).

ASD) in children born between 1992 and 1995 in Staffordshire, United Kingdom. In this population, 96 children were confirmed to have ASD,[25] with 99 percent having received their first MMR vaccine (median age of 13.5 months) and 65.6 percent having received their second MMR vaccine (median age 43.6 months). The investigators compared that sample with two other clinical groups, the Maudsley Hospital Clinic (MHC) and the Maudsley Family Study (MFS) samples. The MHC sample consisted of 68 children with autism born between 1987 and 1996 who had been exposed to the MMR vaccine and had been seen in a clinical setting. The MFS sample consisted of 98 individuals with autism born between 1954 and 1979 seen in a clinical setting, none of whom had been exposed to MMR. All patients were assessed using the standardized ADI, which provided reliable data (e.g., on age at first parental concern, rates of regression) across samples. Data on bowel symptoms and disorders were obtained from the epidemiological (Stafford) survey and immunization records were obtained from computerized records.

The investigators tested all six hypotheses noted above. First, only one child in the epidemiological (Stafford) sample had CDD, resulting in a very low prevalence of CDD (0.6/10,000 [95% CI, 0.02-3.6/10,000]). This is consistent with previous studies and does not suggest an increase in this form of autism in samples of children vaccinated with MMR. In a second analysis, there was no difference across three samples (two MMR-exposed [Stafford and MHC] samples and the one unexposed [MFS] sample) in the mean age at which parents first became concerned about autistic symptoms in their child ($F_{2,250} = 0.02$; not significant). In a third analysis, investigators compared the rates of regression in the two samples for which information on regression was available to see whether the rate of regression increased. The results showed no difference in the rates of regression in the epidemiological sample of 96 children (Stafford sample) who had been exposed to MMR as compared to unexposed comparison group ($X^2 = 3.65$; $df = 2$; p > .15). Fourth, age at parental recognition of first symptoms among children with autism with developmental regression (19.8 months) was similar to that of children with autism without developmental regression (19.3 months). Mean intervals between MMR immunization and parental recognition of autistic symptoms were similar among children with and without regression (248 days versus 272 days; not significant). Finally, in the epidemiologic (Stafford) sample, where data on GI symptoms were available, such symptoms were reported in 18.8 percent of the sample. There was no association between regression and GI symptoms in this study population (OR: 0.63; 95% CI, 0.06-3.2; not significant). The investigators concluded that their study does not support a new phenotype of MMR-induced ASD with features of regression and bowel symptoms.

---

[25]The authors excluded one child with Rett's syndrome.

This study was limited by the use of samples from two different time periods and was thus susceptible to bias caused by secular changes in the diagnostic methods and referral patterns for autism (Wilson et al., 2003). However, these limitations should not affect the inferences regarding regression and bowel symptoms.

United Kingdom. DeWilde and colleagues (2001) conducted a case-control study of children in the United Kingdom to examine whether a temporal association between MMR vaccine and autism existed. The authors hypothesized that onset of developmental regression following MMR vaccine would be reflected in the increased consultations with the child's general practitioner. The Doctor's Independent Network, a general practice database, was used to examine whether children who were subsequently diagnosed with autism had more frequent consultations following MMR vaccine than children who were not vaccinated. Seventy-one children with ASD and 284 matched controls (4:1) were identified during the time period 1989 to 2000. Controls were matched for age, sex, month of MMR vaccination, and general practitioner practice. The authors found no significant difference in consultational behavior between the patients with autism and controls. Furthermore, only one case of ASD was diagnosed within 6 months of MMR vaccination (median time was 1,053 days). A significant limitation of this study is that it included *any* consultation rather than only consultations specific to autism (Wilson, 2004).

Denmark. Madsen and colleagues (2002) conducted a population-based retrospective cohort study comparing the rates of ASD among children in Denmark who were vaccinated with MMR with those who did not receive the MMR vaccine. Study subjects included all children in Denmark born between 1991 and 1998. The cohort was established using data from the Danish Civil Registration system, which assigns a unique identification number to each live birth. This unique identification number is used to link an individual's record with all other national registries.

MMR vaccination status was obtained from data reported to the Danish National Board of Health (NBH) by general practitioners, who administer all MMR vaccinations in Denmark and who are reimbursed for these vaccinations upon reporting them to the NBH. The MMR vaccine was introduced in Denmark in 1987 and was the same vaccine that was used in the United States at the time.[26] Single antigen measles virus has not been used in Denmark. The Danish national vaccine program recommends vaccinating children with MMR at 15 months and 12 years of age and provides the vaccine free of charge. No changes to the MMR

---

[26]The vaccine contained the following vaccine strains: Moraten (measles), Jeryl Lynn (mumps), and Wistar RA 27/3 (rubella).

vaccination schedule were made during the study period. The authors obtained information only on the exposure at 15 months because that was the only one relevant to the outcome measurement in this study.

Information on diagnoses of autism was obtained from the Danish Psychiatric Central Register, which contains information on diagnoses received by patients in inpatient psychiatric hospitals and departments and in all outpatient clinics. Over 93 percent of children were treated on an outpatient basis. Diagnoses were based on ICD-10 codes and included all children with autism (ICD-10 code F84.0 and DSM-IV code 299.00) or another ASD (ICD-10 code F84.1-F84.9). Experts in child psychiatry and autism conducted a record review of 40 patients to validate the autism diagnoses. Thirty-seven (92 percent) of these children met the operational criteria for autistic disorder. The three children who did not meet the operational criteria for autistic disorder were classified as having another ASD. Data on birthweight and gestational age and other confounders were also obtained from other national registries.

Children were followed from 1 year of age until a diagnosis of autism, other ASDs, or associated genetic condition,[27] emigration, death, or end of the follow-up period (December 31, 1999), whichever came first.[28] Children were assigned to the unvaccinated group until they received the MMR vaccine. Incidence-rate ratios (referred to as relative risks) for autism and other ASDs in the MMR-vaccinated group compared with the unvaccinated group were analyzed using a log-linear Poisson regression model. Risk estimates were adjusted for potential confounders, including age, sex, calendar period, socioeconomic status, mother's educational level, gestational age, and birth weight.

A total of 537,303 children were included in the cohort and followed for 2,129,864 person-years. A total of 440,655 children (82 percent) received the MMR vaccine for a total of 1,647,504 person-years of follow-up, compared with 482,360 person-years of follow-up for children who did not receive the MMR vaccine. Of these, 316 children were identified with an autistic disorder and 422 with a diagnosis of another ASD. Mean age at time of MMR vaccination was 17 months, and 98.5 percent of vaccinated children received the MMR prior to 3 years of age. The same proportion of boys (82 percent) were vaccinated as were girls.

After adjusting for potential confounders, the relative risk of autistic disorder among vaccinated children compared with unvaccinated children was 0.92 (95% CI, 0.68-1.24) and the relative risk for other ASD was 0.83 (95% CI, 0.65-1.07). There was no association between age at time of MMR vaccination, time since vaccination, and date of vaccination and the developmenta of autistic disorder.

---

[27]Data for children with inherited genetic conditions associated with autism, including tuberous sclerosis, Angelman's syndrome, Fragile X syndrome, and congenital rubella, were censored to improve the homogeneity of the study population.

[28]Follow-up was halted for 5,811 children because of these factors (5,028 for death or emigration).

The results showed that the risk of autism was comparable both in vaccinated and unvaccinated populations. In addition, there was no temporal clustering of autism cases following immunization. Finally, MMR vaccine was not associated with autism or other ASD. The authors concluded that the study provided evidence against a causal association between vaccines and autism.

Finland. Makela and colleagues (2002) conducted a retrospective cohort study to investigate the association between MMR vaccine and several neurological disorders, including autism, among children in Finland.[29] The study examined two hypotheses: (1) whether there was a clustering of cases of hospitalization for autism after receipt of the MMR vaccine; and (2) whether any recipients of the MMR vaccine who were diagnosed for autism were also hospitalized with inflammatory bowel disease.

In Finland, MMR vaccination at ages 14 to 18 months and 6 years began in 1982. Researchers obtained vaccination records from a national vaccine surveillance study conducted between 1982 and 1986. The register contained records for approximately 86 percent of all children scheduled to be vaccinated between 1982 and 1986. Of the enrolled vaccinees, 535,544 children were 1 to 7 years old at time of the vaccination. Vaccination data on these children was linked with data from the national hospital register. Three hundred fifty-two of them were hospitalized with an autism diagnosis (defined by ICD 8 or 9 codes). Of these, 309 were hospitalized for autism following their MMR vaccination.

Because of the lack of a specific risk period for autism following vaccination, the authors assessed whether there were changes in the overall number of hospitalizations for autism after MMR vaccination for the study as a whole. They found no clustering of hospitalizations for autism following vaccination. Intervals between MMR vaccination and hospitalizations for autism ranged from 3 days to twelve and a half years. Hospitalizations for autism remained relatively stable for the first 3 years and then increased as the child aged, as expected. In addition, of the children hospitalized with autism, none were hospitalized for inflammatory bowel diseases from 1982 to 1995. The authors concluded that the results showed no association between MMR vaccination and autism.

The primary limitation of this study was that it relied only on hospitalization records and thus was unable to identify individuals who were not hospitalized but rather seen on an outpatient basis. While the authors stated that it is common in Finland for children with autism to be admitted to the hospital for observation and testing, a diagnosis of autism does not always involve hospitalization.

Japan. Takahashi and colleagues (2003) conducted a case-control study of children with autism in the Tokyo area growing up between 1988 and 1992 to

---

[29]Although multiple neurological outcomes were studied, for purposes of this report only the autism outcome is discussed.

assess the association of autism with MMR vaccine compared to monovalent measles, mumps, and rubella immunization. From 1989 to 1993, the Japanese national immunization program recommended that MMR vaccine or monovalent measles vaccine be given at age 12 months. Monovalent mumps and monovalent rubella vaccines were optional for children not receiving MMR.

Twenty-one children (4 female, 17 male) with autism were enrolled as cases in the study. Diagnosis of autism was made based on DSM-IV criteria. Physicians from a specialized psychiatric facility in the Tokyo area requested that caregivers of ASD patients born between 1988 and 2000 give consent to release records (response rate with informed consent was 87.5 percent). A control group of 8 females and 34 males (twice the size of the case group) was selected from the same birth year cohort of children who were attending one of the two pediatric clinics in Tokyo. Controls were randomly selected; only those who did not have neuropsychiatric disorders and whose guardian's had consented to disclosure of their records were enrolled in the study (response rate 58 percent). Immunization history data, including information on adverse events, were collected from records contained in the Maternal and Child Health handbook. Completeness of immunization in the case group versus the control group was 90.5 percent versus 100 percent for measles, 42.9 percent versus 78.6 percent for mumps ($p < 0.01$), and 52.3 percent versus 83.3 percent for rubella ($p < 0.01$). Only two cases and four controls received the monovalent measles, mumps, and rubella shots.

The authors used a 1:2 sex-adjusted logistic regression to analyze data collected from the records. Using MMR immunization as a reference, the ORs for the development of ASD were significantly increased for monovalent measles (OR = 5.33; 99% CI, 1.03-27.74), nonmumps immunization (OR = 8; 99% CI, 1.33-48.2), and nonrubella immunization (OR = 8.57; 99% CI, 1.30-56.4). The odds for development of ASD after receipt of monovalent vaccines (mumps and rubella vaccines), compared to the odds of ASD after receipt of the MMR vaccine, were not statistically significant (monovalent mumps: OR = 3.33; 99% CI, 0.45-24.6; monovalent rubella: OR = 3.82; 99% CI, 0.59-24.7). The results suggest a decreased risk of developing autism following MMR compared to monovalent measles, mumps, and rubella vaccines.

The study was limited by the small sample size (N = 21), the potential bias resulting from the informed-consent process,[30] and the poor response rate from the control group, all of which may have exaggerated the findings of no association.

Ecological Studies

United States. Dales and Colleagues (2001) examined trends in autism and MMR immunization coverage among young children in California to determine

---

[30]For instance, the informed-consent process may have discouraged parents of children with a poor immunization history from enrolling their children.

whether a correlation exists. Data on age at first MMR immunization for children born between 1980 and 1994 who were enrolled in California kindergartens was derived from annual reviews of a sample of school records (approximately 600-1,900 children per year). The California Department of Developmental Services provided data on regional service-center caseloads for children born between 1980 and 1994 and having an ICD-9 diagnosis of autistic disorder, which excludes other pervasive developmental disorders.

The authors observed a substantial increase in autism caseloads for successive birth cohorts but relatively stable immunization rates at ages 17 or 24 months. They concluded that these data did not support an association between MMR immunization and an increase in the incidence of autism.

The authors note that data from the California Department of Developmental Studies were not designed to measure trends in autism incidence because other system factors can affect caseloads from year to year. Several methodological limitations in these data have been cited, including the failure to account for changes over time in the population size or composition, in diagnostic concepts, in case definitions, or in age of diagnosis (Fombonne, 2001c). Thus, trends in autism caseload must be interpreted with caution. The authors noted that they were unable to link individual immunization and autism records for the same children. In addition, the data did not provide precise breakdowns of the percentage of children who received the MMR vaccine versus separate administration of monovalent or other combinations of measles, mumps, and rubella vaccines. Historical information suggests though that separate administration was rare in the United States during the period of study.

United States. Geier and Geier (2004a) examined the hypothesized association between MMR vaccine and autism. The number of children with autism was based on data from the DOE regarding children with autism who were enrolled in special education programs. Autism cases were based on the DOE's definition of autism and data collection standards.[31,32] The authors estimated the number of children who developed autism for the birth cohorts in each of the following

---

[31]Every year, the DOE prepares a report for Congress, as mandated by the IDEA, the federal law that supports special education and related services for children and youth with disabilities. The report contains information about many aspects of the IDEA program, including characteristics of the students served, programs and services, and policies. Data have been collected since 1976. Early data were collected by age group rather than by individual age year. Autism was added as a disability category per the 1990 amendments to IDEA. Autism was an optional disability category for federal reporting for 1991-1992 and became a required category in 1992-1993. Prior to the introduction of the autism category in 1990, IDEA served students with autism, but for reporting purposes they were included in a different disability category. (Online. Available at: http://www.ideadata.org/docs/bfactsheetcc.doc.)

[32]The number of autism cases in the special educational system was obtained from the 1999, 2000, and 2003 DOE reports.

years: 1982, 1985, and 1991-1996. They estimated the prevalence of autism in each birth cohort by dividing the number of children with autism in each year by the number of live births that year, using data from the CDC's yearly live birth surveillance data. The number of measles-containing vaccines administered in each respective birth cohort was based on CDC estimates of primary pediatric measles-containing vaccine coverage for birth cohorts in 1982 (67 percent coverage), 1984 (61 percent), 1991 (82 percent), 1992 (82.5 percent), 1993 (84.1 percent), 1994 (90 percent), 1995 (87.8 percent), and 1996 (90.5 percent). The authors plotted the estimated number of primary pediatric measles-containing vaccinations versus the prevalence of autism for each birth cohort examined. The authors reported a slope of 4831[33] and a linear regression coefficient of 0.91.[34] The authors concluded that a potential positive correlation exists between primary pediatric vaccines and autism prevalence.

This study has serious methodological limitations, similar to the other studies by these authors. First, the data on autism cases comes from the DOE dataset, which has significant limitations. As noted previously, these data are based on children with a diagnosis of autism who receive special education services, which may or may not reflect the true prevalence of autism. Furthermore, the child count is a cross-sectional (i.e., point-in-time) count of students served and the appropriateness of the authors' transformation of the cross-sectional autism-caseload data into birth-cohort prevalence data is questionable (Fombonne, 2001a). Changes in either states' policies or IDEA's reporting practices can affect the caseload numbers from year to year. For instance, autism caseload may vary from year to year as the result of policy changes, such as changes to the states' eligibility criteria for particular disabilities. Similarly, prior to the addition of the autism category in 1990, IDEA served students with autism, but for reporting purposes they were reported in a different disability category (see http://www.ideadata.org/docs/bfactsheetcc.doc).

Furthermore, the exposure is not specific to MMR; that is, the data do not provide information on the percentage of children who received the MMR vaccine versus separate administration of monovalent or other combinations of measles, mumps, and rubella vaccines. Finally, the regression model was not described in the paper. The description of analytical methods was not transparent and important details were omitted. As a result, the results of this study are uninterpretable and therefore noncontributory to causality.

United Kingdom. Kaye and colleagues (2001) used population-based data from the U.K. GPRD to conduct a time-trend analysis for estimating changes in the risk of autism and specifically for assessing the temporal relationship between

---

[33]The reported slope of 4831 seems anomalous.

[34]It is unclear whether the authors intended the term "linear regression coefficient" to refer instead to the coefficient of determination (R-sq). Slope (or partial slope) and coefficient are generally interchangeable terms in the context of regression.

MMR vaccination in the United Kingdom and the incidence of autism. The authors noted that the GPRD has been used for numerous published studies and is considered to be complete with respect to vaccination records.

From GPRD records, 305 cases of autism in children aged 12 or younger and diagnosed between 1988 and 1999 were identified. Of these cases, 83 percent were male and 81 percent were referred to a specialist for evaluation of the diagnosis. The estimated annual incidence of diagnosed autism had increased sevenfold from 0.3 per 10,000 person-years in 1988 to 2.1 per 10,000 person-years in 1999, with a median age at first recorded diagnosis of 4.6 years. The authors performed further analyses to estimate the 4-year risk of diagnosed autism for each annual birth cohort. These analyses were restricted to 114 boys born between 1988 and 1993 who were first diagnosed with autism between 2 and 5 years of age. The prevalence of MMR vaccination was calculated separately for each annual birth cohort (restricted to children who were registered with the GPRD within 60 days of birth and had at least 2 years of recorded follow-up).

The 4-year risk of autism increased nearly fourfold from 8 per 10,000 person-years in 1988 to 29 per 10,000 person-years in 1993, while the prevalence of MMR vaccination remained constant, at 97 percent. The authors hypothesized that if MMR vaccine were a major cause of the increasing incidence of autism, then the risk of autism in successive birth cohorts would be expected to stop rising within a few years of the vaccine being widely used. However, because the incidence of autism among 2- to 5-year-olds increased markedly from 1988 to 1993 while MMR vaccine coverage remained over 95 percent for successive birth cohorts, the authors concluded that the results did not support a causal association between MMR vaccination and the risk of autism.

The authors noted they did not review full clinical records for the children diagnosed with autism; such a review would be necessary to provide a more detailed characterization of these children and their diagnosis and to explore other possible explanations for the increase in the observed incidence of autism during the past decade.

Sweden. In a brief commentary, Gillberg and Heijbel (1998) reanalyzed data from a population study of autism conducted in the late 1980s in Sweden (Gillberg et al., 1991). A total of 55 children were diagnosed with autistic disorder based on DSM-III-R criteria, and an additional 19 individuals met criteria for atypical autism based on ICD-10 criteria. The MMR vaccine was introduced into Sweden for 18-month-old children in 1982, and coverage soon rose to above 90 percent. The authors divided the subjects into two groups according to era of birth, as a proxy for exposure to the MMR vaccine: children born between January 1, 1975, and June 30, 1980 (pre-MMR), and children born between July 1, 1980, and December 31, 1984 (post-MMR). The authors hypothesized that if autism were associated with MMR vaccination, children born since July 1980, who were 18 months or younger at the time of MMR introduction, would be at increased risk of having developed autism.

The analysis indicated that 47 of the children (34 with autistic disorder, 13 with atypical autism) were born during the earlier period, and 27 (21 with autistic disorder, 6 with atypical autism) were born during the later period. Because the numbers in the later period were much lower than expected had there been a strong effect at the population level of MMR on the prevalence of autism, the authors concluded that this study did not support the hypothesized association between MMR vaccine and autism. One limitation of this study was that children born from 1980 through 1984 did not have the same length of follow-up as those born earlier, with the maximum follow-up age of 4 for those born in 1984. Although most cases of autism are diagnosed prior to this age, if there was some age dependency in the MMR effect, this study would have been unable to detect it.

This and the other ecological studies are limited in that secular trends in the methods for diagnosing autism may confound any finding of an association or lack of an association. In addition, the ecological study design precludes drawing inferences about individuals based on population data (Wilson et al., 2003).

Studies of Passive Reporting Data

United States. Geier and Geier (2003c) examined reports of serious neurologic symptoms to VAERS following primary pediatric MMR immunization in comparison to reports of these outcomes following DTwP vaccination, which they designated as a control group. The serious neurologic symptoms examined in this study included cerebellar ataxia, autism, mental retardation, and permanent brain damage. The authors used data on vaccine doses distributed per year from the CDC's BSS as a proxy for vaccines administered each year. They used CDC estimates of percent vaccine coverage of each yearly birth cohort from 1994 to 2000. The authors calculated incidence rates[35] for the adverse events, which were then used to calculate the relative risk, attributable risk,[36] and percent associa-

---

[35]The epidemiologic measure "incidence rate" is used incorrectly in this study. An incidence rate is the number of new cases occurring in a defined time period among the population at risk. VAERS cannot be used to calculate incidence rates because the VAERS database does not have complete reporting of all adverse events and because many report events lack a confirmed diagnosis or confirmed attribution to vaccine (Varricchio et al., 2004). Therefore, the numerator for an incidence rate, the number of new events, is incomplete. Further, VAERS does not provide the denominator, that is the population at risk of the event or, in this case, the number of persons vaccinated with the vaccine of interest in the same time period.

[36]The epidemiologic measure "attributable risk" is used incorrectly in this study. As noted by Mann (2003), attributable risk is intended to be a measure of the absolute, rather than the relative, difference in risk among the exposed and unexposed groups. Geier and Geier (2003c) calculate attributable risk by subtracting 1 from the relative risk value (RR−1 = attributable risk). Making attributable risk a fraction of the relative risk provides no information on the absolute or actual risk of thimerosal, nor does it provide information on the proportions of disease either among the exposed or population that can be attributed to exposure.

tion.[37] For autism, they reported a relative risk of 5.2, an attributable risk of 4.2, and a percent association of 84; the statistical significance was p < 0.001, and the 95% CI was 3.0-9.2. The authors report that the serious neurological outcomes were "statistically significantly increased following primary MMR vaccination in comparison to DTwP vaccination" (p. 205).

This study has many of the same methodological limitations as the authors' papers examining thimerosal and autism including the following: using VAERS data to infer causality, failure to clearly delineate the unit of analysis (individual vs. group), inappropriate use of epidemiologic measures (incidence rate and attributable risk), and nontransparent analyses. These problems are discussed in detail in the thimerosal causality section. The study's significant methodological limitations make it results uninterpretable, and therefore noncontributory with respect to causality.

Finland. In 1982 the Finnish National Board of Health and National Public Health Institute launched a long-term MMR vaccination program aimed at the elimination of measles, mumps, and rubella from Finland (Patja et al., 2000; Peltola et al., 1998). All children were to be vaccinated twice with MMR, between the ages of 14 and 18 months and at 6 years. In addition to the primary target groups, intermediate age groups were vaccinated in catch-up programs, unvaccinated adolescents were vaccinated during outbreaks, and adult groups at increased risk of exposure to these diseases (e.g., defense workers, health care workers) were also vaccinated. The live-virus MMR vaccine produced by Merck & Co., Inc. (West Point, PA) was primarily used, except in 1992-1996, when 2,570 doses of Trivirten (Swiss Serum and Vaccine Institute, Bern) were administered to individuals with severe hypersensitivity. Vaccine coverage was around 95 percent, with almost 3 million doses distributed and approximately 1.8 million vaccinations by 1996.

Following introduction of MMR, a countrywide passive surveillance system, based on reporting by health care personnel, was established to gather information about the incidence and nature of all severe adverse events following MMR vaccination. A potentially serious adverse event was one that met at least one of three criteria: (1) a potentially life-threatening disorder (e.g., anaphylaxis); (2) a chronic disease (e.g., rheumatoid arthritis, diabetes) that possibly had been triggered by vaccination; or (3) hospitalization for reasons possibly attributable to MMR vaccine. If an event occurred, a report was filed by health care personnel. The first part of a two-part form was sent immediately, with a serum sample if possible. The second part of the form was completed 2 to 3 weeks later and sent with a second serum sample. Reports were evaluated and contacts were made with the hospital or health center treating the vaccinated person if more informa-

---

[37]Percent association is not a recognized epidemiological measure.

tion was needed. The authors noted that passive surveillance systems may lead to underreporting, and that active surveillance may more reliably detect adverse events. However, awareness of this potential problem prompted organization of an extensive campaign to encourage health care workers and the public to thoroughly report serious events.

From 1982 through 1996, a 14-year surveillance period, adverse events were reported for 437 vaccinations, and 173 events were considered serious according to the criteria noted above. Age at the time of vaccination ranged from 13 months to 23 years. The interval from MMR vaccination to onset of symptoms ranged from a few minutes to 80 days, with peaks during the first 24 hours and at 7 to 10 days. These cases were grouped into several categories: death, likely allergic reactions, neurologic disorders, and miscellaneous reactions. The neurologic disorders included febrile seizures, epilepsy, undefined seizure, encephalitis, meningitis, Guillain-Barré syndrome, gait disturbance, and confusion during fever.

Patja and colleagues (2000) reviewed all 173 serious adverse events reported during this period. Of these, there was one death, 73 cases (42 percent) of likely allergic reactions, 77 cases (45 percent) of neurologic disorders, and 22 cases (13 percent) of miscellaneous reactions. Peltola and colleagues (1998) followed up surveillance-system reports on 31 children, aged from 1 year 2 months to 13 years at vaccination, who developed gastrointestinal symptoms, all except one after the first vaccine dose. Hospital or health records were reviewed, or local public health nurses were interviewed. The interval between the reported event and follow-up ranged from 16 months to over 15 years (median 10 years and 8 months). Neurological symptoms originally reported in these 31 children in-cluded febrile seizures (five cases), headache (two cases), and ataxia (one child).

During the 14 years of MMR vaccination surveillance, no cases of ASD were reported or identified during the follow-up of the 31 children for whom GI disorders were reported following vaccination. Similarly, no cases of ulcerative colitis, Crohn's disease, or any other chronic disorder affecting the GI system were reported. The authors conclude that there is no evidence to support the hypothesis of an association between MMR vaccine and ASD or inflammatory bowel disease.

This study is of limited value to causality because it relies on a passive-surveillance system. Furthermore, the authors found no cases of autism among the 1.8 million vaccinees, a rate that is well below the normal incidence of autism, thereby suggesting a potential reporting bias (Wilson et al., 2003).

Case Series

United Kingdom. Wakefield and colleagues (1998) examined 12 children (11 males, 1 female), aged between 3 and 10 years, consecutively referred to the pediatric gastroenterology department of the Royal Free Hospital and School of Medicine in London. These children each had a history of normal development followed by a loss of acquired skills, including language, and of intestinal symptoms (diarrhea, abdominal pain, bloating, and food intolerance).

Eleven subjects were found to have chronic or acute and chronic nonspecific colitis (non-Crohn's disease or ulcerative colitis). Eight of the 12 subjects were reported to have reactive ileal lymphoid hyperplasia, with 3 of them also having colonic lymphoid hyperplasia, and 1 subject had just colonic lymphoid hyperplasia alone. In addition, nine of the subjects were found to have lymphoid nodular hyperplasia of the terminal ileum. Urinary methylmalonic-acid excretion was significantly elevated in eight children who were tested. The authors reported that there was no clear correlation between the endoscopic appearances and the histologic findings, although none of the findings from the 12 subjects were seen in a series of five ileocolonic biopsies from age-matched and site-matched controls with normal mucosa. In a later study, Wakefield and colleagues (2000) further examined the endoscopic and histopathological features of patients with developmental disorders and bowel symptoms. The cohort of 60 children included the 12 described above.

The authors reported the following behavioral diagnoses for 10 of the children they examined: "autism" for eight subjects; "autism? disintegrative disorder?" for one subject; and "autistic spectrum disorder" for one subject. Two subjects were diagnosed with "post-vaccinial encephalitis?" or "post-viral encephalitis?" The methods used to assess behavioral problems were not clearly stated.

Parents or doctors identified the MMR vaccine as the exposure that was linked to the onset of behavioral problems in six of the eight subjects with definitive autism and in the subject with suspected "post-vaccinial encephalitis." The other two subjects diagnosed with autism had received MMR vaccine, but no specific exposure was linked to the onset of behavioral symptoms. Recurrent otitis media was the exposure identified for the subject with ASD; this subject had previously received MMR vaccine. Measles infection was the identified exposure in the subject with suspected "post-viral encephalitis"; this subject also had previously received MMR vaccine. For the subject with a diagnosis of either autism or disintegrative disorder, the MMR vaccine was linked to deterioration in behavior, and this subject was also reported to have shown slowed development following an earlier exposure to monovalent measles vaccine.

The time between suspected exposure and first clinical and behavioral symptoms ranged from 24 hours to 2 months, with a median of 1 week. Of the eight subjects for whom MMR had been identified as the exposure linked to the onset of behavioral problems, five had early adverse reactions (fever, rash, convulsions). Self-injury behavior was reported for three subjects; gaze avoidance (n = 2), repetitive behavior (n = 1) and loss of self-help (n = 1) were also reported. One subject was reported to have had recurrent viral pneumonia for 8 weeks following vaccination. For the 11 of the 12 subjects for whom age at onset was reported, the range in age at onset of first clinical and behavioral symptoms was 12 months to

4.5 years, with a median of 15 months. The age at first bowel symptoms was reported for 6 of 12 subjects and ranged from 18 to 30 months, with a median of 19 months.

Although these findings may identify a GI condition in a set of children diagnosed with ASD, or showing symptoms of ASD, who received MMR vaccine, they are uninformative in assessing the hypothesized causal association between MMR vaccine and autism and subsequent studies have not been able to replicate or prove this hypothesis. It is difficult to identify a specific time of onset of developmental and GI problems in young children because of the overlap in timing between the typical age at which ASD symptoms are initially suspected and the schedule for MMR and other vaccinations. In addition, given the relatively high vaccine coverage rates, many children with such problems will have received the MMR vaccine within months of the onset of symptoms.

Causality Argument

Studies examining the association between MMR and autism (see Table 10), including nine controlled observational studies (DeStefano et al., 2004; DeWilde et al., 2001; Farrington et al., 2001; Fombonne and Chakrabarti, 2001; Madsen et al., 2002; Makela et al., 2002; Takahashi et al., 2003; Taylor et al., 1999, 2002), three ecological studies (Dales et al., 2001; Gillberg and Heijbel, 1998; Kaye et al., 2001), and two studies based on a passive reporting system in Finland (Patja et al., 2000; Peltola et al., 1998), consistently showed no association. Two studies reported findings of a positive association between MMR and autism. The first was an ecological study (Geier and Geier, 2004a) that reported a potential positive correlation between the number of doses of measles-containing vaccine and the cases with autism reported to the special education system in the 1980s. The second was a study using passive reporting data by the same authors (Geier and Geier, 2003c) that reported a positive correlation between autism reports in the VAERS and estimated administered doses of MMR. However, these two studies are characterized by serious methodological flaws and their analytic methods were nontransparent, making their results uninterpretable, and therefore noncontributory with respect to causality (see text for full discussion). The case-series study by Wakefield and colleagues (1998), which originally raised the hypothesis linking MMR and autism, is uninformative with respect to causality and subsequent studies have not been able to replicate or prove this hypothesis. **Based on this body of evidence, the committee concludes that the evidence favors rejection of a causal relationship between MMR vaccine and autism.** This conclusion is consistent with the finding in the committee's previous report on MMR and autism (IOM, 2001a).

Biological Mechanisms

Autism is a very complex disorder. A strong genetic component clearly exists, but there is a growing understanding that environmental factors might be important contributors to the expression of that genetic susceptibility. Animal models (primarily rat models), clinical observations, and pathological data point to an array of pathways by which autism could possibly develop, though none are proven. Many different pathways might lead to similar expressions, which could account for the multiple presentations of autism.

A link between vaccine components, such as the measles vaccine-strain virus or the ethylmercury preservative thimerosal, is difficult by establish because of the early stage of scientific understanding about the cause(s) of autism. The committee read, and heard presentations at their workshop, about several hypotheses. Data presented to support these hypotheses derive from rodent models of human autism, observations of abnormalities in children with autism or their families, and *in vitro* studies.

One hypothesis about the MMR vaccine involves the presence of measles virus lodging in the intestine of some children and the release of gut-brain mediators (such as opioid peptides) or toxins, leading to autism (Wakefield et al., 2002). Another hypothesis related to MMR vaccine is that children with autism have immune abnormalities that are indicative of vaccine-induced-CNS, immune-mediated damage that leads to autism (Singh, 2004).

The thimerosal-related hypothesis posits that some genetically susceptible children react to the thimerosal in vaccines with increased accumulation and decreased excretion of mercury from the brain, which alters several key biochemical pathways—for example, apoptosis and DNA metabolism—leading to autism (Bradstreet, 2004). A genetically susceptible subset of children who develop autism following vaccinations is one theoretical explanation for the findings in epidemiological studies of no association between vaccination and autism.

MMR Vaccine and Vaccine-Strain Virus in the Intestine

As discussed in a previous portion of this report, a case series published in 1998 described an unusual pathology, ileal lymphonodular hyperplasia, in the intestines of 12 children with developmental disorders, some of whom were described as being autistic (Wakefield et al., 1998). Subsequent work of that laboratory identified the measles virus genome in the ileal lymphoid tissue of 75 out of 91 developmentally disabled children and of 5 out of 70 developmentally normal control children (Uhlmann et al., 2002). Unpublished work by some of those same investigators reported the presence of measles virus F-gene in the cerebral spinal fluid (CSF) of three children with autism in whom MV genome had been previously detected in biopsies of lymphoid nodular hyperplasia (presumably these were subjects in the previously described paper) (Bradstreet, 2004; Sheils et al., 2002). Two of the three children had detectable anti-myelin basic protein (MBP) and measles virus antibodies in the CSF and all three children had detectable serum anti-MBP antibodies. Furthermore, the authors claim that the MV genome was consistent with vaccine strain. However, the specificity of the assay used for indicating vaccine-strain has been questioned (Parks, 2001; Salisbury, 2004; Sheils et al., 2002). A transcript from a court proceeding in the United Kingdom submitted to the committee suggests that strain identity as consistent with vaccine could not be confirmed by other laboratories in the three cases and that virus was absent from three cases not described in the submitted paper (Salisbury, 2004).

Nonetheless, a previous report of this committee concluded that studies documenting the presence of measles virus in the gut of children with autism are not directly relevant to the arguments (causal argument or biological mechanisms argument) regarding vaccine-based adverse events. Even if the measles virus in the gut of some developmentally disabled children were vaccine-strain (which is questionable), it would remain a matter of conjecture that the connection were causal. It is equally likely that autism leads to behaviors (e.g., abnormal eating patterns that lead to intestinal distress) or is associated with other conditions (e.g., immune deficiency) by which measles virus (vaccine-strain or wild-type) hones to altered intestines. Moreover, the finding of measles particles in the gut is not specific to individuals with NDDs; they are also found in neurologically intact individuals with severe bowel disease. Thus, the presence of virus could be secondary to autism or the bowel disease, not a predisposing or causal factor.

The implications of this work for the treatment of children with autism should not be lost in the controversies over the MMR vaccine. If some developmentally disabled children have a previously unrecognized intestinal pathology causing distress, pain, and a cycle of diarrhea and constipation, treatment could lead to a better quality of life and possibly to behaviors conducive to better learning. This could lead to very important advances in the medical and behavioral management of autism. An ongoing study that attempts to replicate the findings of ileal lymphonodular hyperplasia and viral presence in children with autism (described in a subsequent section of this report) might shed light on the role of intestinal disease in autistic manifestations.

Immune Dysregulation

A large number of studies have suggested that immune dysregulation occurs in autism (Korvatska et al., 2002; Krause et al., 2002). Decreased lymphocyte responsiveness in the lymphocyte blastogenesis assay to PHA, ConA, and Pokeweed mitogen has been reported in people with autism as compared with controls (Stubbs and Crawford, 1997; Warren et al., 1986). A study by Warren et al. of 31 autistic patients and 23 healthy control subjects showed that about 40 percent of the patients with autism had significantly reduced natural killer (NK) cell activity (Warren et al., 1987). Gupta et al. noted a decreased proportion of IFN-gamma- and IL-2 (Th1 cytokine)-staining CD4+ T cells in the serum of children with autism compared with healthy controls (Gupta et al., 1998). In contrast, IL-4-(Th2 cytokine)-staining CD4+ T cells were significantly increased in autism. The authors thus suggested an imbalance of Th1 and Th2 like cytokines in autism with consequent depressed cell-mediated immunity in autism. However, the proportion of CD4+ T cells that stained other Th2 cytokines such as IL-6 and IL-10 were not different between the two groups, making it unlikely that a simple Th1-to-Th2 shift had occurred. Moreover, it is difficult to interpret the physiological relevance of differential intracellular cytokine staining of a mixed population of lymphocytes with a whole range of antigenic specificities. Evaluating for Th1/Th2 imbalance is generally more appropriate when considering T cells with a particular antigenic specificity.

In contrast to the abovementioned study, several papers have reported increased levels of plasma IFN-gamma and IL-2 (Th1 cytokines) in people with autism as compared to healthy controls (Singh, 1996; Singh et al., 1991). Increased production of serum IL-12, IL-6, tumor necrosis factor-alpha and IFN-gamma, and increased urinary neopterin have also been reported in people with autism (Croonenberghs et al., 2002; Singh, 1996), suggestive of a generalized activation of the immune system. Consistent with this, Jyonouchi et al demonstrated that PBMCs (peripheral blood mononuclear cells) from patients with autism, both at baseline and after stimulation with LPS (lipopolysaccharide) and PHA (phytohemagluttinin), secreted significantly more pro-inflammatory cytokines (TNF-alpha, IL-1beta, and IL-6) than those from healthy controls and normal siblings (Jyonouchi et al., 2001).

Other groups have shown hypergammaglobulinemia in people with autism, with the IgG2 and IgG4 subclasses being particularly elevated (Croonenberghs, 2002). Increased IgE levels have been reported by some groups in people with autism (Gupta et al., 1996), but the physiological relevance of this is unclear, as atopy is not increased in autism. IgA deficiency has also been reported in autism. In summary, although several studies have reported abnormalities of components of the immune systems, they have often had contradictory results, making it difficult to achieve a consensus on any specific immune abnormality that might characterize autism. More fundamentally, it is not clear how these abnormalities might explain the CNS defects in autism or whether they could be secondary to GI or other complications of developmental disability.

A large number of serum autoantibodies have been detected at a higher frequency in children with autism compared to controls. The antigens against which these autoantibodies are directed include a number of CNS antigens, such as myelin basic protein and neuron-axon filament protein, but they also include a whole host of other proteins, such as nerve growth factor, serotonin receptor, alpha-2-adrenergic receptor, tubulin, heat shock protein 90, and chondroitin sulfate (Connolly et al., 1999; Cook et al., 1993; Evers et al., 2002; Singh et al., 1988, 1993, 1997; Todd and Ciaranello, 1985; Vojdani et al., 2002). Antibodies to chlamydia pneumonia, streptococcal M protein, tubulin, and milk butyrophilin have also been found at increased levels in children with autism compared to controls. This suggests that rather than there being a specific antibody response to CNS antigens, generalized hypergammaglobulinemia resulting from polyclonal B cell activation occurs in autism. Of note in the abovementioned studies, these antibodies were all also found in the serum of healthy controls, albeit at lower levels—i.e., they were not specific to autism, making their pathogenic significance questionable.

A study by Comi et al. highlighted the association of autism with autoimmune disorders in the patients' relatives (Comi et al., 1999). In this study, 46 percent of patients with autism had two or more family members with autoimmune disorders, compared to 26 percent of controls. The most common autoimmune disorders in both groups were type I diabetes, adult rheumatoid arthritis, hypothyroidism, and systemic lupus erythematosus. The increase in familial autoimmune disorders suggests a possible link, in some genetically susceptible families, between autoimmunity and autism. Of note in this study, however, is that there was no increase in the incidence of autoimmune disease in the patients with autism themselves. A major criticism of this study is that it was retrospective and thus suffered from recall bias. As stated by the authors, the families of children with autism were more likely to exhaustively assess the medical histories of all their relatives to look for a reason for their child's autism. Similar findings of family history of autoimmune disorders were reported by Sweeten et al. (2003), but were not found in another study (Micali et al., 2004).

Several autoimmune disorders have known linkage to particular major histocompatibility complex (MHC) haplotypes. An association of autism with the MHC has been reported, with an increased frequency of the extended haplotype B44-SC30-DR4 in people with autism, their mothers, or both (40 percent) as compared to controls (2 percent) (Daniels et al., 1995; Warren et al., 1992). The null allele of the C4B complement protein gene and the third hypervariable region (HVR-3) of certain DRB1 alleles, both known to be part of the ancestral haplotype B44-SC30-DR4, also are associated with autism (Warren et al., 1991, 1996). Although the possession of such a haplotype may deleteriously affect antigen presentation to lymphocytes and have immunological consequences, it is also possible that another nonimmune related gene linked to or contained within this extended MHC haplotype is more relevant to the development of autism by, for example, modifying synaptic plasticity. The relevance of this MHC haplotype is thus unclear.

Torrente et al. reported additional possible evidence for autoimmunity in autism, in the form of immune-mediated enteropathy (Torrente et al., 2002). Through immunohistochemistry, the authors demonstrated extensive lymphocyte infiltration in both the epithelium and lamina propria of the small intestine in children with regressive autism (23 out of 25 patients) compared to normal controls and patients with cerebral palsy. Epithelial IgG and complement C1q deposition was also seen in 23 out of 25 children with autism, and not seen in the other groups. It was suggested that this autoimmune enteropathy may lead to altered cognitive functioning through failure to detoxify neuroactive substances originating from the gut. In other studies, ileal lymphoid hyperplasia and lymphocytic colitis, with striking infiltration of CD8 and T cells, have been reported in children with regressive autism (Wakefield et al., 1998, 2000). It should be pointed out that these GI studies have all been in children with regressive autism, which is an uncommon[38] subtype of autism. It is thus difficult to know how these findings apply to the majority of people with autism. More importantly, it is not clear whether the autism is the cause or the consequence of the GI abnormalities.

Although a number of studies have suggested immune dysregulation in autism, there is as yet no evidence that these findings are directly related to the pathogenesis of autism. Unlike what is known about neuroimmunological disorders that affect the brain, such as multiple sclerosis and acute disseminated encephalomyelitis, there is no evidence of immune activation or an inflammatory process within the autistic brain. Neuropathological studies of autism have revealed no evidence of cerebral inflammatory lesions or microglial activation, which is a common feature in immune-mediated encephalitis (Bauman and Kemper, 1997). However, there are very few autopsy studies of brains from people with autism and this has not been fully investigated. Analysis of CSF from young children with autism, including screening for sensitive inflammatory markers such as quinolinic acid and neopterin, has also found no evidence of inflammation (Comi et al., 1999). The sample size in these studies is small, however.

As mentioned, autoantibodies to cerebral antigens, including MBP, have been found at higher titers in children with autism compared to controls. It is important to note, however, that these studies all evaluated serum and *not* CSF or brain tissue. Furthermore, it should be realized that not all autoantibodies are pathogenic—indeed, they are found in healthy individuals with no evidence of autoimmune disease. Some of the factors that determine the pathogenicity of a particular autoantibody include its affinity or avidity of binding to the autoantigen, its access to the autoantigen, and its ability to fix, complement, and facilitate cell-mediated death. With respect to the pathogenicity of serum anti-MBP antibodies in people with autism, no signs of demyelination have been found either on MRI or neuroanatomically in children with autism (Rumsey and Ernst, 2000). It is thus debatable how relevant serum anti-MBP antibodies may be to the pathogenesis of autism. It is not clear whether the dysregulation precedes the autism or is part of the syndrome.

Some investigators have tried immunotherapies, such as corticosteroids and intravenous immunoglobulin, in people with autism on the assumption that immune

---

[38]Estimates of the proportion of autism that is of the regressive type range from 0 to 40 percent.

dysfunction plays an important role in the etiology of autism. There have been anecdotal reports both of treatment success and treatment failure (DelGiudice-Asch et al., 1999; Gupta et al., 1996; Plioplys, 2000). In any event, regardless of the results of these studies, they cannot be used to conclusively determine the importance of the immune system in autism pathogenesis, as they were not done in a double blind, placebo-controlled (i.e., nonbiased) fashion and did not use standardized behavioral tests as outcome measures.

It is clear that genetics plays a strong role in the etiology of autism. There is a 90 percent concordance rate in monozygotic twins and 5-10 percent concordance in same-sex dizygotic twins (Bailey et al., 1995; Ritvo et al., 1989). In addition, the rate of autism among the siblings of an affected child is 3-6 percent, which is 50-100 times higher than in the general population (Rutter, 1999). The significant sibling risk versus the rapid falloff in the risk for distant relatives is consistent with the involvement of multiple susceptibility genes.

Rett's syndrome, which is in the same family of pervasive developmental disorders as autism, is characterized by a course of symptoms and regression that are analogous to some children with autism (Zoghbi, 2003). The regression is seen after about a year of normal development. It was recently discovered that Rett's syndrome is caused by mutations (mainly *de novo*) in the methyl-CpG-binding protein 2 (MECP2) gene (Amir et al., 1999). Rett's syndrome thus provides an example of dynamic and altered brain development in a genetically determined condition. MECP2 specifically binds methylated DNA and functions as a general transcriptional repressor (Nan et al., 1998). MECP2 mutations are thought to result in at least a partial loss of function by altering the normal developmental regulation of imprinted genes, some of which are responsible for the specific neurologic phenotype of Rett's syndrome. Immune dysregulation similar to that described in autism, such as immunological abnormalities in T cells and decreased activity of natural killer cells, has been noted in Rett's syndrome (Fiumara et al., 1999). This raises the possibility that MECP2 mutations, in addition to causing the neurodevelopmental abnormality that characterizes Rett's syndrome, also cause immune abnormalities. By analogy to Rett's syndrome, similar epigenetic mechanisms may be operating in autism that simultaneously lead to abnormal development in the immune and central nervous systems (Zimmerman, 2000). However, the deviations from expected levels in various *in vitro* laboratory assays in both these conditions may represent only a secondary effect of the developmental or behavioral abnormalities.

Thimerosal and Autism

Abnormal Mercury Metabolism

The hypotheses about thimerosal and autism involve aspects of mercury kinetics in children. As described in the beginning of this report, when all recommended childhood vaccines contained thimerosal as a preservative, infants could have been (and most certainly many were) exposed to levels of ethylmercury that exceeded the safety standards for methylmercury exposure set by two of three major governmental agencies (EPA and ATSDR). Recent publications describe measurements of mercury burden in children with autism and controls (Bradstreet et al., 2003; Holmes et al., 2003), and although these studies do not directly address the issue of thimerosal exposure through vaccination, the authors posit that children with autism have an abnormal metabolic response to mercury burden.

Two primary approaches, mercury levels in hair and responses to chelation, have been used. Hair samples from 94 children with autism and 45 control children were analyzed for mercury levels (Holmes et al., 2003). These hair samples were described as "first haircut" samples, and the authors suggest that they reflect mercury exposures during gestation and infancy. The median age at time of hair sampling was 17.7 months for the population with autism and 17.8 months for the controls. Mercury levels were assayed by a commercial laboratory using plasma mass spectroscopy. Children were assigned by observation into severe, moderate, or mild autism severity. Maternal exposures to amalgams, Rho D immunoglobulin injection (which at the time contained thimerosal), and fish consumption during pregnancy were assessed. The vaccination history of the child was also documented.

Mercury levels in these "first haircut" samples were significantly lower in the children with autism than in the controls. Subgroup analysis showed decreasing mercury levels in the hair as the autism severity score increased. (The severity score was based on observations during a clinical encounter; it does not appear to be derived from a standard diagnostic tool.) The mothers of children with autism had higher exposures to Rho D immunoglobulin and slightly more amalgam fillings than did the mothers of controls. Mercury levels in the hair of control children increased with the number of amalgams in the mother, maternal fish consumption, and childhood vaccinations, whereas there was no similar pattern in children with autism.

However, the hair sample is described as "first baby haircut," with median age of just under one and a half years of age and not the infant hair at birth. Thus the implications of the mercury measurements for prenatal exposures is unclear. Other concerns are the biased sampling. The clinical practice from which the case children were derived is specifically interested in the role of vaccines in autism and the control children were solicited via the internet and newsletters related to autism. Only 9 percent of the control mothers received RhoGAM, when national statistics suggest that 15 percent of women are Rh negative (Warren Grant Magnuson Clinical Center, National Institutes of Health, 2004). The types of fish consumed were not elaborated, nor were enough details of the hair samples given to indicate the period of the infant's life the hair sample represented. Further, infant exposures to other sources of mercury postnatally were not ascertained. The relevance of prenatal exposures through the mother to this hair analysis was unclear, unless the assumption was that the mother's mercury burden is passed on to the infants through breastfeeding, which was not controlled for. The authors interpreted these findings as suggesting that children with autism do not excrete mercury into the hair—i.e., that the mercury burden remains bioactive within the body. Direct evidence for this hypothesis was not presented.

A second, related line of inquiry involves the results of chelation. A recently published study examined mercury excretion upon chelation challenge of children with autism compared to controls (Bradstreet et al., 2003). The controls were healthy children whose parents sought chelation therapy in response to their worries about heavy metal toxicity. Children with autism (n = 221) excreted significantly more mercury in the urine upon chelation challenge than controls (n = 18). Cadmium and lead concentrations were not different between controls and children with autism. However, the range of mercury excreted was 0 to 59 with a mean of 4.1 (micrograms mercury per gram creatine) and a standard deviation of 8.6, suggesting that the data might be skewed in the direction that many if not most of the children with autism are excreting little mercury.

One treatment center has conducted preliminary clinical studies suggesting defective functioning of metallothionein (MT) in patients with autism. Abnormal levels of blood copper and zinc were detected in 499 of 503 patients with autism (Walsh, 2001). The authors hypothesized that autism might be caused by a genetic defect in MT or by a biochemical abnormality disabling MT. Because MT is involved in detoxification of heavy metals such as mercury, the authors suggested that this genetic defect might make the patients more susceptible to thimerosal exposures. Another investigator submitted preliminary data to the committee regarding defective functioning in children with autism of trans-sulfuration pathways that are involved in generating the antioxidant peptide glutathione (James, 2004, unpublished data).

The authors of the first two studies hypothesized that some children with autism have an inherent inability to excrete mercury (thus the low levels of mercury in their hair) and consequently accumulate more in the body (which is then excreted at high levels upon chelation challenge). According to this hypothesis, thimerosal is just a source of mercury, which some children with autism cannot process, leading to higher mercury burdens and to more adverse reactions to thimerosal than are experienced by nonautistic children. An analogous clinical condition might be Wilson's disease, a genetic inability to handle copper (Aposhian, 2004). Similarly, abnormalities in lead metabolism and clinical toxicity have been linked to genetic variation in aminolevulinic acid dehydratase (Smith et al., 1995). However, similar variations in mercury metabolism have not been identified.

An observational study of stool, blood, and urine mercury levels following vaccination was conducted. The authors suggest that administration of thimerosal-containing vaccines does not raise blood mercury concentrations above safe levels (Pichichero et al., 2002). Mercury concentrations were low in urine after vaccination but were high in stools of thimerosal-exposed 2-month-olds (mean 82 ng/g dry weight) and in 6-month-olds (mean 58 ng/g dry weight). Estimated blood half-life of ethylmercury was 7 days (95% CI, 4-10 days). The authors concluded that ethylmercury seems to be eliminated from blood rapidly via the stools after vaccination with TCVs. However, peak blood levels of mercury shortly after vaccination were not measured in this study, which might be more relevant to considerations of toxicity. Others have used the data in that paper to estimate that the peak blood mercury level in one infant could have surpassed established safety levels[39] (Halsey and Goldman, 2001).

Preliminary findings from nonhuman primates suggest that thimerosal accumulates in the blood and brain of developing nonhuman primates to a much lower degree than does methylmercury (Sager, 2004). If humans respond to thimerosal more or less as this animal model does, it seems unlikely that thimerosal accumulates to toxic levels following vaccination. However, the laboratory animals had no background mercury exposures, whereas recent CDC estimates are that 8 percent of women aged 16 to 49 years of age have elevated blood mercury levels (Schober et al., 2003). The same dataset was used to estimate that over 300,000 newborns each year in the United States may have been exposed to methylmercury at levels higher than that determined to be without adverse effect (Mahaffey et al., 2004). Thus, it is possible that the amount of mercury that accumulates in the brain following thimerosal could be additive to the exposures from other sources. Thus, the contribution of vaccine-related mercury to total mercury burden and toxicity is unclear. If altered mercury metabolism in a small subset of children vaccinated with TCV were responsible for autism, it would be very difficult to detect in experimental studies. However, the relevance of the kinetic data to the question of autism is unclear, as autism has not been shown to be associated with mercury exposure.

Apoptosis

Several investigators have explored the possibility that autism is associated with altered apoptosis, the cellular pathway of programmed cell death that is important in brain development, among other physiological processes. This has been a subject of interest because of histological findings in autistic individuals' brains of altered cerebellar purkinje cells, although a definitive role for altered apoptosis in these alterations is not established. Postmortem tissue from people with autism and matched controls has been used to measure markers of Bcl-2, a regulatory protein shown to prevent apoptosis and that has also been shown to be

---

[39]The reader is referred to previous sections of the report that discuss the guidelines for mercury exposure. In addition, it should be mentioned that the guidelines do not establish a safe exposure level, rather they indicate a level of exposure below which no adverse effects have been detected.

reduced in schizophrenic brains. One study found decreased Bcl-2 levels in autistic cerebella, suggesting a vulnerability to pro-apoptotic stimuli and to neuronal atrophy as a consequence of decreased removal of other cell types (Fatemi et al., 2001). Another study from the same laboratory reported decreases of Bcl-2 and increases of p53, also related to apoptosis, in the parietal cortex, superior frontal cortex, and cerebellar cortex of people with autism compared to matched control brain tissues (Araghi-Niknam and Fatemi, 2003). However, there is currently no evidence that such abnormalities are causally related to the development of autism. These biochemical alterations could as likely be secondary to the cause of autism.

Studies show effects of thimerosal on apoptosis in cell culture. Incubation of cultured human frontal cortex (from patients with seizure disorder), fibroblasts, and Jurkat cells (T-cell lymphoblasts) with thimerosal led to DNA damage, nuclear membrane damage, caspase 3 activation, and apoptotic morphology (Baskin et al., 2003). Jurkat cells were incubated with thimerosal in another study, leading to apoptosis, and reduced intracellular glutathione (Makani et al., 2002). Caspase 3 is an enzyme activated in apoptosis. In an extension of that work, lymphocytes taken from children with autism, and from their unaffected siblings as controls, were immortalized and exposed to thimerosal (unpublished data; Baskin, 2004). In 3 of 10 pairs of cell cultures (from cases and matched control), the samples from the child with autism showed increase in caspase 3 expression and decreases in an assay of general metabolic activity and calcine-AM esterase activity. A known neurotoxin, thimerosal has many effects in cell culture (see following section), but the relevance of these findings to a causal pathway in autism is theoretical. The absence of changes in caspase 3 expression in the majority (7 of 10) of cell culture-pairs suggests these biochemical pathways are not necessarily relevant to the expression, let alone the cause, of autism.

Methylation Pathways

Methionine synthase (MS) is an enzyme that is involved in the conversion of homocysteine to methionine. Such methylation is involved in many enzymatic pathways, including gene regulation; methylation of DNA, for example, modulates gene expression and the integrity of DNA. A recently published paper reported a new finding that dopamine and insulin-like growth factor-1 (IGF-1) stimulate methionine synthase activity and folate-dependent methylation of phospholipids in cultured human neuroblastoma cells (Waly et al., 2004). Dopamine is a neurotransmitter associated with movement, attention, memory, and many other brain functions. IGF-1 has been shown to have anti-apoptotic effects in many cells, including oligodendrocytes (those cells responsible for myelination in the brain). The authors also reported that several known neurotoxins, including thimerosal, ethanol, lead, and aluminum, inhibited these effects of dopamine and IGF-1. The authors hypothesize that disruption of this pathway by thimerosal leads to autism, ADHD, and other developmental disorders. However, the committee is aware of no evidence that autism is caused by alterations in this biochemical pathway. In addition, the evidence that several important toxicants disrupt this pathway and that it is involved in many physiological effects weakens the argument that thimerosal might cause autism through this mechanism.

Rodent Models of Autistic-like Pathology and Behavior

Three rodent models of autism-like behaviors and neuropathology have been developed. Two of the models involve infection at an early age with an infectious agent and the development of behavioral, pathological, and neurochemical abnormalities that the investigators construe as similar to autism. The third model uses thimerosal as the environmental trigger of results that are similar but not identical to the infectious models. None is as yet completely described. The thimerosal model is as yet unpublished.

The bornavirus model of autism was reviewed in the first report of the committee (IOM, 2001a). Neonatal rats infected with bornavirus develop abnormal behaviors that might be analogous to behavior expressed by children with autism, including hyperactivity, impairments in righting reflex, and abnormal play behavior (Carbone et al., 2002; Hornig et al., 1999). Histological examination shows damage to the granule cells of the dentate gyrus and cerebellar Purkinje cells. Other abnormalities include reduced (less complex) branching of some hippocampal neurons and other evidence of alterations in a components of the glutamate neurotransmitter pathway in the hippocampus (Hornig, 2004).

Increased mRNA levels for pro-apoptotic proteins (Fas, caspase-1), decreased mRNA levels for the anti-apoptotic bcl-x, and in situ labeling of fragmented DNA implicate a role for apoptosis in the cell loss. Although inflammatory infiltrates are observed transiently in frontal cortex, glial activation persists for several weeks in concert with increased levels of proinflammatory cytokine mRNAs (interleukins 1alpha, 1beta, and 6 and tumor necrosis factor alpha) and progressive hippocampal and cerebellar damage (Hornig et al., 1999).

Another rodent model of infection-mediated neuronal and behavioral abnormalities is the group A beta-hemolytic streptococcal (GABHS) model, which is being used to study a relatively new syndrome, pediatric autoimmune neuropsychiatric disorder associated with streptococcal infection (PANDAS). Behavioral manifestations of PANDAS include obsessive-compulsive disorder and tics (Swedo et al., 1998). Children with PANDAS have an increased incidence of some of the immunological and neurochemical laboratory abnormalities (e.g., evidence of antibrain autoantibodies) compared with children who have likely had the same streptococcal infection but did not develop neuropsychiatric disease (Pavone et al., 2004). Injection of an inactivated GABHS in mice leads to abnormal behavior and immunoglobulin staining in the brain (Hornig, 2004).

A similar rodent model using ethylmercury exposure is under development by the same laboratory (Hornig, 2004).[40] Investigators dosed mice in a manner intended to be analogous in time and dose to the U.S. childhood immunization schedule. Strains with differing sensitivity to autoimmune reactions were used. The SJL strain of mice reacted to the thimerosal administration differently than did four less-reactogenic mouse strains. The mice were said to display differences in weight gain, to exhibit mutilation behaviors, and to have destruction of the CA3 region of the hippocampus, increased cell density in other parts of the hippocampus and dentate gyrus, and enlarged brains. Although this model uses thimerosal and is possibly more relevant to the discussion at hand, it assumes that autism is caused by an autoimmune reaction. A previous section discussed the lack of evidence of autoimmune-mediated CNS damage in the brains of patients with autism.

The relevance of rodent models, including the three described above, is difficult to assess because the rodent "clinical" endpoints may not reflect the human ones, because there is limited understanding of the etiology of autism, and because the methods used to cause changes in the animals may bear no relationship to pathogenesis of the human disease. The committee accepts that under certain conditions infections and heavy metals, including thimerosal, can injure the nervous system. These rodent models are useful for understanding some of the processes by which these exogenous agents may exert their damage. However, the connection between these models and autism is theoretical.

Genetic Susceptibility

Despite legitimate concern about vaccine safety, few dispute the fact that adverse reactions to vaccines are rare, leading some to claim that infants and young children will not experience adverse reactions unless they possess some unusual characteristic that increases susceptibility—in particular, a genetic predisposition. This suggestion has currency now because of the discovery of genetic variants in humans that do indeed change the way individuals react to certain medications, a field of research known as pharmacogenetics. For example, Factor V Leiden deficiency, a genetic variant present in up to five percent of the population, increases susceptibility to blood clotting. Some have suggested that individuals be tested for Factor V Leiden deficiency before using hormones, oral contraceptives, or other drugs that are known to increase blood clotting. Another example is an enzyme, CYP2C9, that metabolizes warfarin, a medication commonly used for blood thinning. One percent of the U.S. population is

---

[40]This study was released on June 8, 2004, as a *Molecular Psychiatry* advance online publication entitled *Neurotoxic effects of postnatal thimerosal are mouse strain dependent* (http://www.nature.com/), which occurred after the Immunization Safety Review Committee released their report. However, Dr. Hornig presented the unpublished results of this study to the Committee on February 9, 2004.

deficient in this enzyme, and thus requires only a fraction of the normal dose of warfarin. Some have argued that patients should be tested for this enzyme before treatment with warfarin in order to avoid the risk of overdose with the drug.

These and other examples can be used to hypothesize that something similar might be operating in infants and young children exposed to certain vaccines or vaccine components. This hypothesis cannot be excluded by epidemiological data from large population groups that do not show an association between a vaccine and an adverse outcome. Depending upon the frequency of the genetic defect, a rare event caused by genetic susceptibility could be missed even in large study samples.

Some researchers working in pharmacogenetics believe that this area of research will eventually explain many of the variations in outcomes currently observed in medical practice. Others are skeptical. The committee recognizes this line of reasoning as a theoretical explanation for the data presented in this report but has found no corroborating data in the laboratory, in animals, or in humans linking vaccines or vaccine components to autism based on genetic susceptibility.

Biological Mechanisms Argument

Autism is a heterogeneous disorder with a broad range of behavioral symptoms and severity. As yet, a biological marker specific for autism has not been defined. It is thus possible that autism encompasses a spectrum of disease subtypes that have different etiologies. This could explain the wide range of immunological abnormalities that have been found in the serum of patients with autism, with some studies reporting evidence of decreased cell-mediated immunity (CMI), and others reporting increased/overactive CMI. The evidence presented for an association of autoimmunity with autism is the report that autoimmune enteropathy was seen in a large proportion of subjects with "regressive autism." This effect is purported by some to be a clinical subtype of autism, making it difficult to extrapolate this finding to the majority of patients with autism. Other support for an association of autism with immune dysfunction includes reports of increased frequency of an extended MHC haplotype in autism, increased autoantibodies to brain antigens, and an increased incidence of autoimmune diseases noted in a retrospective study of relatives of people with autism.

However, despite evidence of immune dysregulation in the serum of people with autism, there is as yet no evidence that the immune system plays a role in the neuropathogenesis of autism. Unlike neuroimmunological diseases such as multiple sclerosis, there is no evidence of immune activation or inflammatory lesions in the brains or CSF of people with autism. Furthermore, wild-type measles infection is associated with a variety of very serious CNS damage, but it has never been associated with autism. The lack of such evidence also argues against a causal link with MMR vaccination.

It is clear from twin and family studies that there is a strong genetic basis for autism. The recent discovery of the genetic basis of Rett's syndrome, a pheno-typically similar NDD with similarly described laboratory immunological abnor-malities, may shed some light on the pathogenesis of autism. Similar epigenetic mechanisms in autism may lead to combined abnormal development of the CNS and immunologic irregularities.

The hypotheses reviewed by the committee were that vaccine-induced au-tism represents the end result of a combination of susceptibilities (possibly ge-netic) to immune dysfunction or to abnormal mercury metabolism. Posited inter-mediate steps include enzymatic abnormalities that might be related to apoptosis or cellular signaling, leading to an array of behavioral, cognitive, sensory, and motor disturbances. Other environmental exposures could have similar effects. Demonstrating an adverse effect of Hg *in vitro* does not readily translate into a physiologic argument. These processes are widespread in the body, so that the argument why these adverse effects cause autism must also include how the effects occur in specific tissues at specific times in development to cause the symptoms of autism, and do not cause more widespread dysfunction. No theory explains why vaccination would be the only environmental cause of these wide-ranging effects. If MMR vaccine or thimerosal is one of many environmental causes of these effects (or if thimerosal is one source of many of mercury expo-sure), without a specific "fingerprint" or "signature" that suggests vaccine or mercury as the causative factor, knowing if MMR or thimerosal is responsible for the adverse effects in an individual case is impossible.

Rodent models suggest that reactions to some infectious agents (e.g., bornavirus and group A streptococcus) lead to somewhat specific neuronal cell death and evidence of autoimmune reactions in the developing and adult brains of rodents. The animals also exhibit abnormal behaviors. These immunological and behavioral findings are similar to those seen in some humans after infection: the behavior in children with PANDAS or in the animal models resembles the behav-ior constellations in children with autism. A similar set of comparisons can be made with mercury exposures (Bernard et al., 2001), although autism has never been documented as a consequence of high-dose mercury exposure, including acrodynia. While analogies are useful for hypothesis generation, they do not substitute for direct evidence.

The committee notes several factors that limit acceptance at this time of the hypothesis that vaccines cause autism. The evidence offered for the hypothesis includes data from *in vitro* experimental systems, analogies between rodent be-havior, and human behavior and clinical observations that are at least as well explained as being comorbid disease expressions than as causal factors. That is, it is possible that some people with autism, perhaps even a subgroup that could eventually be identified by genetic markers, have abnormal immune reactions and abnormal mercury metabolism, but that vaccination of these individuals does not cause these abnormalities or autism itself. However, the experiments showing effects of thimerosal on biochemical pathways in cell culture systems and showing abnormalities in the immune system or metal metabolism in people with autism are provocative; the autism research community should consider the appropriate composition of the autism research portfolio with some of these new findings in mind. However, these experiments do not provide evidence of a relationship between vaccines or thimerosal and autism.

In the absence of experimental or human evidence that vaccination (either the MMR vaccine or the preservative thimerosal) affects metabolic, developmental, immune, or other physiological or molecular mechanisms that are causally related to the development of autism, the committee concludes that the hypotheses generated to date are theoretical only.

SIGNIFICANCE ASSESSMENT

Autism leads to substantial challenges for the families of affected individuals because many people with autism remain dependent throughout their lives. Special education costs can exceed $30,000 per year. The annual cost of care in a residential school may be as much as $80,000-100,000 (CDC, 1999a). In addition to the substantial financial strains, families of children with autism face other demands. During the public session in March 2001 and in the material submitted for the February 2004 meeting, parents described round-the-clock efforts to care for their child, the difficulty of finding knowledgeable and sympathetic health care providers, the challenges in finding high-quality information, and the frustrations of seeing their child change from being active and engaged to being aloof and nonresponsive. Many clinicians, including several committee members, have treated children with autism and witnessed the difficulties and pain experienced by the children and their families.

Although autism is recognized as a serious condition and strides have been made in understanding the disease in many areas, significant gaps remain, particularly regarding etiology and risk factors. These gaps include uncertainty about prevalence and incidence trends; limited knowledge of the natural history of autism, including its early onset and regressive forms; the lack of a strong biological model for autism; the lack of a diagnostic biomarker; limited understanding of potentially associated features (e.g., immune alterations, enterocolitis); and no current basis for identifying possible subtypes of autism with different pathogeneses related to genetic and environmental interactions. Research has been hindered by changing case definitions and the heterogeneity of study populations that may include cases linked to other known medical risk factors (e.g., Fragile X).

Vaccine-preventable disease can also result in significant burden to individuals, families, and society. The introduction of vaccines has brought dramatic reductions in the incidence of vaccine-preventable diseases. For example, prior to the introduction of the measles vaccine in the United States in 1963, an average of 400,000 measles cases were reported each year (CDC, 1998). Since most children acquired measles, this number is likely to be a serious underestimate, attributable to underreporting and other factors. A more accurate estimate of measles incidence prior to 1963 is probably 3.5 million to 4 million cases per year, essentially an entire birth cohort (CDC, 1998). One analysis suggests that the 4 million cases of measles per year in the United States resulted in the following complications per year: 150,000 cases of respiratory complications, 100,000 cases of otitis media, 48,000 hospitalizations, 7,000 instances of seizures, and 4,000 cases of encephalitis (Bloch et al., 1985). Using the incidence rate of 4 million cases per year and the measles case fatality rate of 1.0-2.0 deaths per 1,000 cases (CDC, 1998), an estimated 4,000-8,000 deaths would have occurred annually from measles complications.

With the measles, mumps, and rubella vaccines available, diseases prevented by these vaccines have declined and vaccine coverage rates have increased. Measles cases decreased to 22,000-75,000 per year through the late 1970s (CDC, 1998). During the period from 1981 to 1988, following the introduction of the current MMR vaccine, there were generally fewer than 5,000 cases per year, but the number rose to almost 28,000 cases in 1990 during a serious measles outbreak (Atkinson et al., 1992; CDC, 1998). By 1993, however, with renewed immunization efforts, transmission of indigenous measles in the United States almost disappeared (Watson et al., 1998). In 1999, only 100 cases of measles were reported, and a majority of these were imported or import-linked cases (CDC, 2000). By 2000, measles was no longer considered endemic in the United States (CDC, 2000). In 2003, only 42 cases of measles were reported in the United States (CDC, 2004).

A combined MMR vaccine was originally introduced in 1971 and replaced by the current MMR vaccine in 1979. By 1998, MMR vaccination coverage had reached its highest level ever, with an estimated 92 percent of children aged 19-35 months vaccinated (CDC, 2000). The coverage estimate for 2000 is slightly lower, at 91 percent (CDC, 2002). With coverage rates at this level, it means that each year about 3.4 million children aged 12-24 months receive the MMR vaccine.

The hypothesis that vaccines, specifically MMR vaccine and the preservative thimerosal, cause autism is among the most contentious of issues reviewed by vaccine safety committees of the IOM. One needs to read just one of the many websites and internet-based discussion groups on the issue of autism[41] to get a picture of the complicated lives of families with children with autism and the anger of some families toward the federal government (particularly the CDC and FDA), vaccine manufacturers, the field of epidemiology, and traditional biomedical research. The volume of correspondence to the committee on this issue is impassioned and impressive. There are, however, little data to shed light on how many families believe that vaccination actually caused their child's autism, [42] so

---

[41] See http://health.groups.yahoo.com/group/Autism-Mercury/messages.

[42] Over three thousand families have filed claims for compensation for autism with the Vaccine Injury Compensation Program (VICP).

that the magnitude of concern in the general population is uncertain. **However, the committee concludes that because autism can be such a devastating disease, any speculation that links vaccines and autism means that this is a significant issue.**

There are many examples in medicine of disorders defined by a constellation of symptoms that have multiple etiologies, and autism is likely to be among them. Determining a specific cause in the individual is impossible unless the etiology is known and there is a biological marker. Determining causality with population-based methods such as epidemiological analyses requires either a well-defined at-risk population or a large effect in the general population. Absent biomarkers, well-defined risk factors, or large effect sizes, the committee cannot rule out, based on the epidemiological evidence, the possibility that vaccines contribute to autism in some small subset or very unusual circumstances. However, there is currently no evidence to support this hypothesis either.

As we have learned more about the causes of autism, some cases have been reclassified as other conditions—for example, Rett's syndrome. Additional etiologies are likely to be identified. However, as of yet, the vast majority of cases with autism cannot be consistently and accurately subclassified. Thus, if there is a subset of individuals with autism syndrome triggered by exposure to vaccines, our ability to find it is very limited in the absence of a biological marker. The committee has yet to see any convincing evidence that supports the theory that vaccines are associated with an increase in the risk of autism, either to the population at large or to subsets of children with autism. Although this area of inquiry is interesting, it is only theoretical. However, interactions between genetic susceptibility and environmental triggers are being studied across a broad spectrum of disorders, the cause of which is not understood. Different expressions of the ASD spectrum could arise from the same or different exposures. These relationships could be a source of important new understanding of this family of disorders.

While the committee strongly supports targeted research that focuses on better understanding the disease of autism, from a public health perspective the committee does not consider a significant investment in studies of the theoretical vaccine-autism connection to be useful at this time. The nature of the debate about vaccine safety now includes a theory that genetic susceptibility makes vaccinations risky for some people, which calls into question the appropriateness of a public health, or universal, vaccination strategy.[43] However, the benefits of

---

[43]There are, of course, populations at risk for some very specific vaccine adverse events. For example, people with severe immunosuppression are at risk for developing vaccine-associated paralytic polio and the inactivated vaccine has long been recommended for those people. However, the current debate implicates as yet undefined susceptibilities (not proven to exist) to a host of serious and less well-defined adverse outcomes, such as neuroimmunological brain damage.

vaccination are proven and the hypothesis of susceptible populations is presently speculative. Using an unsubstantiated hypothesis to question the safety of vaccination and the ethical behavior of those governmental agencies and scientists who advocate for vaccination could lead to widespread rejection of vaccines and inevitable increases in incidences of serious infectious diseases like measles, whooping cough, and Hib bacterial meningitis.

The committee urges that research on autism focus more broadly on the disorder's causes and treatments for it. Thus, **the committee recommends a public health response that fully supports an array of vaccine safety activities. In addition the committee recommends that available funding for autism research be channeled to the most promising areas.**

The committee emphasizes that confidence in the safety of vaccines is essential to an effective immunization program—one that provides maximum protection against vaccine-preventable diseases with the safest vaccines possible. Questions about vaccine safety must be addressed responsibly by public health officials, health professionals, and vaccine manufacturers. Although the hypotheses related to vaccines and autism will remain highly salient to some individuals, (parents, physicians, and researchers), this concern must be balanced against the broader benefit of the current vaccine program for all children.

RECOMMENDATIONS FOR PUBLIC HEALTH RESPONSE

Specific recommendations regarding policy review, epidemiologic research and surveillance, and communication follow. The committee also revisits and discusses many of the recommendations of its two previous reports on vaccines and autism (IOM, 2001a,b).

Policy Review

• **At this time, the committee does not recommend a policy review of the licensure of MMR vaccine or of the current schedule and recommendations for the administration of the MMR vaccine.**

• **At this time, the committee does not recommend a policy review of the current schedule and recommendations for the administration of routine childhood vaccines based on hypotheses regarding thimerosal and autism.** At the time of the committee's previous report on thimerosal and NDDs (IOM, 2001b), several universally recommended vaccines contained thimerosal. In that report the committee recommended that appropriate professional societies and government agencies give full consideration to removing thimerosal from vaccines administered to infants, children, or pregnant women in the United States. Currently, thimerosal has in fact been removed from all universally recommended childhood vaccines except influenza. A thimerosal-free preservative influenza vaccine exists, however, and is available for use in infants, children, and pregnant women. There are a few vaccines with thimerosal (e.g., Td) that infants and young children[44] could be exposed to, but only under very special circumstances.

• The committee also recommended in its prior report that the appropriate professional societies and government agencies review their policies on the non-vaccine biological and pharmaceutical products that contain thimerosal and are used in infants, children, and pregnant women. The committee's recommendation reflected concern about total mercury burden and potential risk of certain NDDs. The committee believes that these ongoing reviews are important and should continue. At the same time, the committee recognizes that many other countries, particularly developing countries, must rely on multidose vaccine vials that use thimerosal as a preservative. Because thimerosal is an antibacterial agent that has been highly successful in preventing field contamination, its removal from multidose vials would increase the risk of bacterial infection leading to toxic shock syndrome or death. The option of using single dose vaccines, which do not require thimerosal, is not feasible for some countries because of limits in the production of single-dose vaccines and lack of infrastructure for the transportation and storage of single-dose vials in a cold-chain system. While the United States chose to eliminate thimerosal from routine childhood vaccines as a precautionary measure and because it was feasible, the committee recognizes that other countries have different constraints and other factors; their own assessments of the risks and benefits may lead those countries to reach different conclusions regarding the thimerosal content of their vaccines. **Given the lack of direct evidence for a biological mechanism and the fact that all well-designed epidemiological studies provide evidence of no association between thimerosal and autism, the committee recommends that cost-benefit assessments regarding the use of thimerosal-containing versus thimerosal-free vaccines and other biological or pharmaceutical products, whether in the United States or other countries, should not include autism as a potential risk.**

Surveillance and Epidemiologic Research

• **The committee reaffirms its previous recommendation to use standard and accepted case definitions and assessment protocols for ASD to enhance the precision and comparability of results from surveillance, epidemiological studies, and biological investigations. Studies should also address the heterogeneity in the etiology of ASD and the spectrum of clinical presentation.**

• **The committee reaffirms its previous recommendation to conduct clinical and epidemiological studies of sufficient rigor to identify risk factors and biological markers of ASD in order to better understand genetic or environmental causes of ASD.**

---

[44]Td is recommended for children 12-18, but it is conceivable that some infants and young children could receive Td in lieu of DTaP.

Autism is a complex disease with unknown etiology. A number of research studies are being conducted to examine that etiology, as well as brain structure and function, developmental course, epidemiology, and treatment. To evaluate and compare these current and future studies, accepted and consistent case-definition and assessment protocols are critical.

• Currently, adverse events associated with vaccines are monitored through several mechanisms, including the pre-and postlicensure studies undertaken by vaccine manufacturers, the VAERS, and the CDC's large-linked database (LLDB). **Surveillance of adverse events related to vaccines is important and should be strengthened in several ways:**

— The committee recommends that standardized case definitions for adverse events be adopted. The committee notes that the lack of standardized case definition for adverse events following vaccination is a recurring concern for the committee and for all who study immunization safety. The committee thus encourages the work recently begun by the Brighton Collaboration to develop, through an international consensus process, a set of standard definitions for adverse events (brightoncollaboration.org), as well as the work of the newly established Clinical Immunization Safety Assessment centers (www.cdc.gov/programs/immun8.htm).

— The committee recommends that formal guidelines or criteria be developed for using VAERS data to study adverse events. VAERS, the national passive surveillance system administered by CDC and FDA, monitors adverse events following immunization through reports from health care providers, manufacturers, and the public. Reports to VAERS indicate a temporal, but not necessarily causal, relationship between an adverse event and a vaccine. Furthermore, because VAERS data come from a passive reporting system, they are subject to a variety of limitations, including underreporting of adverse events and lack of a representative control group. Although VAERS is of limited utility in assessing causality, it has served as an early warning system for potential adverse events from vaccination (for example, in the case of intussusception and rotavirus vaccine) and as a useful tool for generating hypotheses on vaccine safety that can be investigated in more structured epidemiological studies. Formal guidelines for analyzing these data for studying adverse events are needed, however, to avoid promulgation of misinformation.

— The committee recommends the continued use of large-linked databases, active surveillance, and other tools to evaluate potential vaccine-related adverse events. The VSD project, which was initiated in 1990 as a partnership between CDC and eight large HMOs, is another example of LLDB that is used to monitor vaccine safety. The VSD includes information which covers more than six million people on all vaccines administered within the study population and includes information on vaccine type, vaccination date, concurrent vaccinations, the manufacturer, lot number, and injection site. Data from medical records are then monitored for potential adverse events resulting from immunization. The VSD project has been used, for example, on investigations of adverse events from thimerosal and other hypotheses (http://www.cdc.gov/nip/vacsafe/default.htm#VSD).

— **The committee supports the development of Clinical Immuniza- tion Safety Assessment (CISA) centers to improve understanding of adverse events at the individual level.** While these mechanisms exist for reporting adverse events and conducting epidemiological studies, until recently no coordi- nated facilities existed in the U.S. to investigate or manage adverse events on an individual level. CISA centers are a new initiative designed to improve the scien- tific understanding of vaccine safety at the individual patient level. These centers are a collaboration between CDC and clinical academic centers across the United States that are sources of clinical expertise in evaluating and treating adverse events following immunization. CISA centers will serve as an intermediate step between passive reporting (i.e., providing information on individual cases of adverse events with no or minimal follow-up) and more rigorous epidemiological investigations into vaccine safety, such as the use of LLDBs, clinical trials, and case-control or cohort studies. These centers will systematically evaluate cases of adverse events reported to VAERS, and selected cases will undergo enhanced follow-up and targeted clinical evaluation to better understand the mechanism(s) and risk factors involved. These evaluations will be used to develop clinical protocols and patient management guidelines that can be used by all health care providers. The CISAs will also evaluate groups of patients with similar adverse events, using a standard protocol, in order to elucidate the mechanism(s) by which unusual or severe adverse reactions occur. Through such evaluation, genetic or other risk factors that predispose individuals to these reactions may be determined.

The committee wishes to comment on several of the other recommendations it made in its 2001 report on MMR and autism. First, the committee recom- mended exploring whether exposure to MMR vaccine is a risk factor for ASD in a small number of children. To date, no convincing evidence of a clearly defined subgroup with susceptibility to MMR-induced ASD has been identified. How- ever, genomics and proteonomics could reveal in the future whether or not any genetic susceptibility to vaccine-induced autism exists.

The committee also recommended targeted investigations of whether measles vaccine-strain virus is present in the intestines of some children with ASD. The committee recommended this research because the findings most salient in the public debate over the hypothesized relationship between MMR vaccine and ASD is the case series reported in 1998 (Wakefield et al., 1998). The committee understands that researchers from Columbia University and CDC are currently working with researchers from the original reporting lab to study this issue and that results will be forthcoming. In addition, in the previous report (IOM, 2001a), the committee recommended studying the possible effects of different MMR immunization exposures. For example, the committee noted that studies might enroll children whose families have chosen not to have them receive the MMR vaccine. To date, this type of study has been difficult to do with sufficiently large numbers. One alternative strategy would be to conduct trials in which the MMR vaccine is delayed among some children, so that it does not coincide with administration of TCVs. This option introduces ethical concerns about having insufficient vaccine coverage in the population for herd immunity and about leaving individual children unprotected against measles, mumps, and rubella, diseases which can cause serious complications and are widely prevalent throughout the world.

• Many of the epidemiological research recommendations of the committee's 2001 report on thimerosal and NDDs are either under way or have been completed. Researchers have undertaken a number of case-control studies examining the potential link between NDDs and TCVs, epidemiological studies comparing the incidence and prevalence of NDDs before and after the removal of thimerosal from vaccines, and studies of neurodevelopmental outcomes of children from other countries who did not receive thimerosal-containing doses of DTaP. Insofar as monitoring of ASD occurs, **one area of complementary research that the committee continues to recommend is surveillance of ASD as exposure to thimerosal declines.** Any research in this area should be conducted with critical attention to case definition, diagnostic criteria, and other factors (for example, data collection procedures and definitions of autism in the special education system) that could affect prevalence estimates of ASD. As noted above, thimerosal has been removed from routine childhood vaccines as a precautionary measure. If TCVs are the primary cause for the rise in ASD, as some have argued, then one would expect to see a sharp decline in the incidence of ASD as thimerosal is removed from vaccines and other biological/pharmaceutical products and exposure declines. If rates of ASD continue to increase following the removal of thimerosal, however, then TCVs could not be the primary cause and research efforts on ASD should be redirected to other potential etiological mechanisms.

• Individuals may be exposed to inorganic mercury and mercurial compounds through a variety of sources, including dental amalgams, environmental or occupational exposure, and the consumption of seafood and fish. Based on the literature and presentations at the committee meetings, little is known about the levels of background exposure to mercury in the population. One recent study found that approximately 8 percent of women had concentrations higher than the EPA's recommended reference dose (Schober et al., 2003), suggesting that at least some proportion of the population is at risk for mercury toxicity. **The committee recommends increased efforts to quantify the level of prenatal and postnatal exposure to thimerosal and other forms of mercury in infants, children, and pregnant women.**

Clinical Studies

• The committee heard from some parents of children with ASD who have chosen to rely on chelation therapy as a treatment. Some reported that unaffected siblings of children with ASD have been chelated as well. The committee saw no scientific evidence, however, that chelation is an effective therapy for ASD or is even indicated in these circumstances. Chelation therapy is currently indicated only for high-dose, acute mercury poisonings. Even in these cases, however, chelation therapy has not been established to improve renal or nervous system symptoms of chronic mercury toxicity (Sandborgh Englund et al., 1994) and has had no effect on cognitive function when used for excretion of another heavy metal—lead (Rogan et al., 2001). Because it is unlikely to remove mercury from the brain, chelation is useful only immediately after exposure and before damage has occurred (Evans, 1998). Moreover, chelation therapy has serious risks; for example, some chelation therapies might cause the release of mercury from soft-tissue stores, thus leading to increased exposure of the nervous system to mercury (Wentz, 2000). **Because chelation therapy has potentially serious risks, the committee recommends that it be used only in carefully controlled research settings with appropriate oversight by Institutional Review Boards protecting the interests of the children who participate.**

Communication

Many parents described to the committee their concerns about the MMR vaccine and thimerosal use in vaccines. Many expressed their frustration and difficulties in making informed decisions about vaccination of their children as their level of trust in the government, media, and science in general has declined. One such example of communication problems that led to controversy and animosity over vaccine safety issues was the VSD research regarding TCVs and NDDs. Because of the importance and difficulty of maintaining mutual trust, a model that focuses on increasing public participation in risk decisionmaking is likely to make that process more democratic and improve the relevance and quality of the technical analysis (Slovic, 1999). Such participative processes may not necessarily lead to increased acceptability of risk policies, but may lead to higher quality decision-making processes (Arvai, 2003).

However, better risk-benefit communication requires attention to the needs of both the scientific and public communities. Many scientists need to develop a more comprehensive understanding of what risk-benefit communication entails and the rich knowledge base that can be used to design strategic communication programs. Appreciating that risk-benefit communication requires two-way exchanges of information and opinions (NRC, 1989) and working from a larger frame of communication methods, scientists will be able to work more effectively with the public to address vaccine-related issues. A mix of information, dissemination, education services, and community-based dialogues are probably needed (NRC, 1989).

To address these goals, the committee looked at existing programs that promote dialogue between various stakeholders around issues where science, research, and policy intersect. One innovative model is Project LEAD® developed by the National Breast Cancer Coalition (NBCC), a grassroots advocacy group (Dickersin et al., 2001; Hinestrosa, 2001). This program promotes open communication and exchange of information between consumers, scientists, researchers, and policymakers. It is multifaceted in that it combines both didactic and interactive learning activities with goals such as improving understanding of research, influencing legislation and policy, and conducting outreach. A key tenet of this program is to ensure that breast-cancer activists play an integral role in policy and research decisions, given their unique and critical perspectives on the issues. Scientists also gained a better understanding of advocates' perspectives on the issues and learned from them how to better communicate their findings. (More information can be found by going to the NBCC website at http://www.natlbcc.org/ and clicking on Project LEAD.)

Similarly, the Committee on the Public Understanding of Science (COPUS) was created in 1985 by the British Association, the Royal Institution, and the Royal Society to support and encourage ways of increasing public understanding and access to scientific literature in the United Kingdom. The COPUS Grant Schemes, begun in 1987, are funded and administered by the Royal Society to encourage small-scale science communication activities. The 2003/2004 COPUS Grant Schemes in particular are designed to make science, engineering, and technology available to a broad range of public audiences and to improve communication between scientific communities, professionals, and public audiences about funding priorities. (More information can be found at http://www.copus.org.uk/.)

Another potential model might be the IOM's Vaccine Safety Forum, which was established in 1995 to examine critical issues and discuss methods for improving the safety of vaccines and vaccination programs. Members of the forum included parents or consumer groups with an interest in immunization, individuals representing vaccine manufacturers, physicians, officials from federal agencies responsible for regulating vaccines and implementing vaccine policies, and academic researchers with expertise in vaccine-related issues. The Forum provided an opportunity to convene individuals from a variety of government, academic, industry, and citizen groups for regular and open dialogue. The objective was to identify key issues rather than to resolve them (IOM, Vaccine Safety Forum Workshop Summary).

The committee recommends developing programs to increase public participation in vaccine safety research and policy decisions and to enhance the skills and willingness of scientists and government officials to engage in constructive dialogue with the public about research findings and their im-

plications for policy development. Programs such as Project LEAD®, COPUS Grant Schemes, or the IOM Vaccine Safety Forum may serve as useful models. Any proposed program should be easily accessible to the public and should involve a wide range of individuals. Additionally, ways to rebuild trust between scientists, professionals, media, and government should be explored.

SUMMARY

This eighth and final report of the Immunization Safety Review Committee examines the hypothesis that vaccines, specifically the measles-mumps-rubella (MMR) vaccine and thimerosal-containing vaccines, are causally associated with autism. The committee reviewed the extant published and unpublished epidemiological studies regarding causality and studies of potential biologic mechanisms by which these immunizations might cause autism. The committee concludes that the body of epidemiological evidence favors rejection of a causal relationship between the MMR vaccine and autism. The committee also concludes that the body of epidemiological evidence favors rejection of a causal relationship between thimerosal-containing vaccines and autism. The committee further finds that potential biological mechanisms for vaccine-induced autism that have been generated to date are theoretical only.

The committee does not recommend a policy review of the current schedule and recommendations for the administration of either the MMR vaccine or thimerosal-containing vaccines. The committee recommends a public health response that fully supports an array of vaccine safety activities. In addition, the committee recommends that available funding for autism research be channeled to the most promising areas. The committee makes additional recommendations regarding surveillance and epidemiological research, clinical studies, and communication related to these vaccine safety concerns. Please see Box 2 for a summary of all conclusions and recommendations.

BOX 2
Committee Conclusions and Recommendations

SCIENTIFIC ASSESSMENT
Causality Conclusions

The committee concludes that the evidence favors rejection of a causal relationship between thimerosal-containing vaccines and autism.

The committee concludes that the evidence favors rejection of a causal relationship between MMR vaccine and autism.

Biological Mechanisms Conclusions

In the absence of experimental or human evidence that vaccination (either the MMR vaccine or the preservative thimerosal) affects metabolic, developmental, immune, or other physiological or molecular mechanisms that are causally related to the development of autism, the committee concludes that the hypotheses generated to date are theoretical only.

SIGNIFICANCE ASSESSMENT

The committee concludes that because autism can be such a devastating disease, any speculation that links vaccines and autism means that this is a significant issue.

PUBLIC HEALTH RESPONSE RECOMMENDATIONS

The committee recommends a public health response that fully supports an array of vaccine safety activities. In addition the committee recommends that available funding for autism research be channeled to the most promising areas.

Policy Review

At this time, the committee does not recommend a policy review of the licensure of MMR vaccine or of the current schedule and recommendations for the administration of the MMR vaccine.

At this time, the committee does not recommend a policy review of the current schedule and recommendations for the administration of routine childhood vaccines based on hypotheses regarding thimerosal and autism.

Given the lack of direct evidence for a biological mechanism and the fact that all well-designed epidemiological studies provide evidence of no association between thimerosal and autism, the committee recommends that cost-benefit assessments regarding the use of thimerosal-containing versus thimerosal-free vaccines and other biological or pharmaceutical products, whether in the United States or other countries, should not include autism as a potential risk.

Surveillance and Epidemiologic Research

The committee reaffirms its previous recommendation to use standard and accepted case definitions and assessment protocols for ASD to enhance the precision and comparability of results from surveillance, epidemiological studies, and biological investigations. Studies should also address the heterogeneity in the etiology of ASD and the spectrum of clinical presentation.

The committee reaffirms its previous recommendation to conduct clinical and epidemiological studies of sufficient rigor to identify risk factors and biological markers of ASD in order to better understand genetic or environmental causes of ASD.

Surveillance of adverse events related to vaccines is important and should be strengthened in several ways:

The committee recommends that standardized case definitions for adverse events be adopted.

The committee recommends that formal guidelines or criteria be developed for using VAERS data to study adverse events.

The committee recommends the continued use of large-linked databases, active surveillance, and other tools to evaluate potential vaccine-related adverse events.

The committee supports the development of Clinical Immunization Safety Assessment (CISA) centers to improve understanding of adverse events at the individual level.

One area of complementary research that the committee continues to recommend is surveillance of ASD as exposure to thimerosal declines.

The committee recommends increased efforts to quantify the level of prenatal and postnatal exposure to thimerosal and other forms of mercury in infants, children, and pregnant women.

Clinical Studies

Because chelation therapy has potentially serious risks, the committee recommends that it be used only in carefully-controlled research settings with appropriate oversight by Institutional Review Boards protecting the interests of the children who participate.

Communication

Better risk-benefit communication requires attention to the needs of both the scientific community and public communities. Many scientists need to develop a more comprehensive understanding of what risk-benefit communication entails and the rich knowledge base that can be used to design strategic communication programs. Thus, the committee recommends developing programs to increase public participation in vaccine safety research and policy decisions and to enhance the skills and willingness of scientists and government officials to engage in constructive dialogue with the public about research findings and their implications for policy development.

REFERENCES

AAP (American Academy of Pediatrics) and USPHS (U.S. Public Health Service). 1999. Joint statement of the American Academy of Pediatrics (AAP) and the United States Public Health Service (PHS). *Pediatrics* 104(3 Pt 1):568-9.

Amir RE, Van den Veyver IB, Wan M, Tran CQ, Francke U, Zoghbi HY. 1999. Rett syndrome is caused by mutations in X-linked MECP2, encoding methyl-CpG-binding protein 2. *Nat Genet* 23(2):185-8.

APA (American Psychiatric Association). 1994. *Diagnostic and Statistical Manual of Mental Disorders*. 4th ed. Washington, DC: APA.

APA. 2000. *Diagnostic and Statistical Manual of Mental Disorders; Text Revision*. 4th ed. Washington, DC: APA.

Aposhian HV. 2004. Presentation to the Immunization Safety Review Committee. *A Toxicologist's View of Thimerosal and Autism*. Washington, DC.

Araghi-Niknam M, Fatemi SH. 2003. Levels of Bcl-2 and P53 are altered in superior frontal and cerebellar cortices of autistic subjects. *Cell Mol Neurobiol* 23(6):945-52.

Arvai JL. 2003. Using risk communication to disclose the outcome of a participatory decision-making process: effects on the perceived acceptability of risk-policy decisions. *Risk Anal* 23(2):281-9.

Atkinson WL, Orenstein WA, Krugman S. 1992. The resurgence of measles in the United States, 1989-1990. *Annu Rev Med* 43(6):451-63.

Bailey A, Le Couteur A, Gottesman I, Bolton P, Simonoff E, Yuzda E, Rutter M. 1995. Autism as a strongly genetic disorder: evidence from a British twin study. *Psychol Med* 25(1):63-77.

Ball LK, Ball R, Pratt RD. 2001. An assessment of thimerosal use in childhood vaccines. *Pediatrics*. 107(5):1147-54.

Baskin D. 2004. Presentation to the Immunization Safety Review Committee. Washington, DC.

Baskin DS, Ngo H, Didenko VV. 2003. Thimerosal induces DNA breaks, caspase-3 activation, membrane damage, and cell death in cultured human neurons and fibroblasts. *Toxicol Sci* 74(2):361-8.

Bauman M, Kemper T. 1997. Neuroanatomic observations of the brain in autism. Bauman M, Kemper T, eds. *The Neurobiology of Autism*. Baltimore: Johns Hopkins University Press. Pp. 119-45.

Bernard S, Enayati A, Redwood L, Roger H, Binstock T. 2001. Autism: a novel form of mercury poisoning. *Med Hypotheses* 56(4):462-71.

Bertrand J, Mars A, Boyle C, Bove F, Yeargin-Allsopp M, Decoufle P. 2001. Prevalence of autism in a United States population: the Brick Township, New Jersey, investigation. *Pediatrics* 108(5):1155-61.

Black C, Kaye JA, Jick H. 2002. Relation of childhood gastrointestinal disorders to autism: nested case-control study using data from the UK General Practice Research Database. *British Med J* 325(7361):419-21.

Blaxill M. 2001. Presentation to Immunization Safety Review Committee. *Rising Incidence of Autism: Association with Thimerosal*. Washington, DC.

Bloch AB, Orenstein WA, Stetler HC, Wassilak SG, Amler RW, Bart KJ, Kirby CD, Hinman AR. 1985. Health impact of measles vaccination in the United States. *Pediatrics* 76(4):524-32.

Bradstreet J. 2004. Presentation to the Immunization Safety Review Committee. *Biological Evidence of Significant Vaccine Related Side-effects Resulting in Neurodevelopmental Disorders*. Washington, DC.

Bradstreet J, Geier D, Kartzinel J, Adams J, Geier M. 2003. A case-control study of mercury burden in children with autistic spectrum disorders. *J Am Phys Surg* 8(3):76-9.

Bristol MM, Cohen DJ, Costello EJ, Denckla M, Eckberg TJ, Kallen R, Kraemer HC, Lord C, Maurer R, McIlvane WJ, Minshew N, Sigman M, Spence MA. 1996. State of the science in autism: report to the National Institutes Health. *J Autism Dev Disord* 26(2):121-54.

Burd L, Fisher W, Kerbeshian J. 1987. A prevalence study of pervasive developmental disorders in North Dakota. *J Am Acad Child Adolesc Psychiatry* 26(5):700-3.

California Department of Developmental Services. 2003. *Autistic Spectrum Disorders. Changes in the California Caseload. An Update: 1999 Through 2002.* Sacramento, CA: California Health and Human Services Agency.

California Health and Human Services Agency, Department of Developmental Services. 1999. *Changes in the Population of Persons with Autism and Pervasive Developmental Disorders in California's Developmental Services System: 1987 Through 1998.*

Carbone KM, Rubin SA, Pletnikov M. 2002. Borna disease virus (BDV)-induced model of autism: application to vaccine safety test design. *Mol Psychiatry* 7 (Suppl 2):S36-7.

Casanova MF, Buxhoeveden DP, Switala AE, Roy E. 2002. Neuronal density and architecture (Gray Level Index) in the brains of autistic patients. *J Child Neurol* 17(7):515-21.

CDC (Centers for Disease Control and Prevention). 1991. Hepatitis B Virus: A Comprehensive Strategy for Eliminating Transmission in the United States Through Universal Childhood Vaccination: Recommendations of the Immunization Practices Advisory Committee (ACIP). *Morb Mortal Wkly Rep.* 40(RR-13):1-19 .

CDC. 1997. Measles eradication: recommendations from a meeting cosponsored by the World Health Organization, the Pan American Health Organization, and CDC. *Morb Mortal Wkly Rep* 46(RR-11):1-20.

CDC. 1998. Measles, mumps, and rubella—vaccine use and strategies for elimination of measles, rubella, and congenital rubella syndrome and control of mumps: recommendations of the Advisory Committee on Immunization Practices (ACIP). *Morb Mortal Wkly Rep* 47(RR-8):1-57.

CDC. 1999a. Autism spectrum disorders among children. [Online] Available: http://www.cdc.gov/ncbddd/fact/tasdfs.htm [accessed 2001].

CDC. 1999b. Thimerosal in vaccines: a joint statement of the American Academy of Pediatrics and the Public Health Service. *Morb Mortal Wkly Rep* 48(26):563-5.

CDC. 2000. Measles—United States, 1999. *Morb Mortal Wkly Rep* 49(25):557-60.

CDC. 2002. Estimated vaccination coverage with individual vaccines by 3 months of age by state and immunization action plan area- US, National Immunization Survey Q1/2001-Q4/2001. Available [online]: http://www.cdc.gov/nip/coverage/NIS/01/TAB4-3months_iap.htm [accessed December, 2002].

CDC. 2003a. ACIP expands recommendation for vaccinating children in the 2004-05 flu season. [Online] Available at: www.cdc.gov/flu/professionals/acip/acipchild0405.htm.

CDC. 2003b. Prevention and control of influenza: Recommendations of the Advisory Committee on Immunization Practices (ACIP). *Morb Mortal Wkly Rep* 52(RR-8):1-35.

CDC. 2004. Prevention and control of influenza: Recommendations of the Advisory Committee on Immunization Practices (ACIP). *Morb Mortal Wkly Rep* 53:1-40.

Chen RT. 1994. Special methodological issues in pharmacoepidemiology studies of vaccine safety. Strom BL, ed. *Pharmacoepidemiology.* 2nd ed. New York: Wiley.

Comi AM, Zimmerman AW, Frye VH, Law PA, Peeden JN. 1999. Familial clustering of autoimmune disorders and evaluation of medical risk factors in autism. *J Child Neurol* 14(6):388-94.

Connolly AM, Chez MG, Pestronk A, Arnold ST, Mehta S, Deuel RK. 1999. Serum autoantibodies to brain in Landau-Kleffner variant, autism, and other neurologic disorders. *J Pediatr* 134(5):607-13.

Cook EH Jr, Perry BD, Dawson G, Wainwright MS, Leventhal BL. 1993. Receptor inhibition by immunoglobulins: specific inhibition by autistic children, their relatives, and control subjects. *J Autism Dev Disord* 23(1):67-78.

Courchesne E, Carper R, Akshoomoff N. 2003. Evidence of brain overgrowth in the first year of life in autism. *JAMA* 290(3):337-44.

Croen LA, Grether JK, Hoogstrate J, Selvin S. 2002. The changing prevalence of autism in California. *J Autism Dev Disord* 32(3):207-15.

Croonenberghs J, Wauters A, Devreese K, Verkerk R, Scharpe S, Bosmans E, Egyed B, Deboutte D, Maes M. 2002. Increased serum albumin, gamma globulin, immunoglobulin IgG, and IgG2 and IgG4 in autism. *Psychol Med* 32(8):1457-63.

Dales L, Hammer SJ, Smith N. 2001. Time trends in autism and in MMR immunization coverage in California. *JAMA* 285(9):1183-5.

Daniels WW, Warren RP, Odell JD, Maciulis A, Burger RA, Warren WL, Torres AR. 1995. Increased frequency of the extended or ancestral haplotype B44-SC30-DR4 in autism. *Neuropsychobiology* 32(3):120-3.

Davidovitch M, Glick L, Holtzman G, Tirosh E, Safir MP. 2000. Developmental regression in autism: maternal perception. *J Autism Dev Disord* 30(2):113-9.

Davis R. 2004. Presentation to the Immunization Safety Review. *Review of 'Safety of Thimerosal-Containing Vaccines: a Two Phased Study of Computerized Health Maintenance Organization Databases.'* Washington, DC.

DelGiudice-Asch G, Simon L, Schmeidler J, Cunningham-Rundles C, Hollander E. 1999. Brief report: a pilot open clinical trial of intravenous immunoglobulin in childhood autism. *J Autism Dev Disord* 29(2):157-60.

DeStefano F, Bhasin TK, Thompson WW, Yeargin-Allsopp M, Boyle C. 2004. Age at first measles-mumps-rubella vaccination in children with autism and school-matched control subjects: a population-based study in metropolitan Atlanta. *Pediatrics* 113(2):259-66.

DeWilde S, Carey IM, Richards N, Hilton SR, Cook DG. 2001. Do children who become autistic consult more often after MMR vaccination? *British J Gen Pract.* 51(464):226-7.

Dickersin K, Braun L, Mead M, Millikan R, Wu AM, Pietenpol J, Troyan S, Anderson B, Visco F. 2001. Development and implementation of a science training course for breast cancer activists: Project LEAD (leadership, education and advocacy development). *Health Expect* 4(4):213-20.

Evans H. 1998. Mercury. *Environmental and Occupational Medicine.* 3rd ed. Philadelphia: Lippincott-Raven.

Evers M, Cunningham-Rundles C, Hollander E. 2002. Heat shock protein 90 antibodies in autism. *Mol Psychiatry* 7(Suppl 2):S26-8.

Farrington CP, Miller E, Taylor B. 2001. MMR and autism: further evidence against a causal association. *Vaccine* 19(27):3632-5.

Fatemi SH, Halt AR, Stary JM, Realmuto GM, Jalali-Mousavi M. 2001. Reduction in anti-apoptotic protein Bcl-2 in autistic cerebellum. *Neuroreport* 12(5):929-33.

FDA (Food and Drug Administration). 2001. Thimerosal content in some currently manufactured U.S. licensed vaccines (table). Accessed July, 2001. Web Page. Available at: http://www.fda.gov/cber/vaccine/thimcnt.htm.

FDA. 2004a. VAERS reports of autism. (Email communication from Jane Woo, Food and Drug Administration, March 31, 2004.)

FDA. 2004b. VAERS reports of autism. (Email communication from Jane Woo, Food and Drug Administration, March 2, 2004.)

FDA. 2004c. VAERS reports of autism. (Email communication from Jane Woo, Food and Drug Administration, March 8, 2004.)

FDA. 2004d. Table 1: Technical Review. (E-mail communication from William Egan, Food and Drug Administration, May 11, 2004.)

FDA. 2004e. Thimerosal content in vaccines. (Email communication from Karen Midthun, Food and Drug Administration, May 7, 2004.)

Filipek PA, Accardo PJ, Baranek GT, Cook EH, Dawson G, Gordon B, Gravel JS, Johnson CP, Kallen RJ, Levy SE, Minshew NJ, Ozonoff S, Prizant BM, Rapin I, Rogers SJ, Stone WL, Teplin S, Tuchman RF, Volkmar FR. 1999. The screening and diagnosis of autistic spectrum disorders. *J Autism Dev Disord* 29(6):439-84.

Fiumara A, Sciotto A, Barone R, D'Asero G, Munda S, Parano E, Pavone L. 1999. Peripheral lymphocyte subsets and other immune aspects in Rett syndrome. *Pediatr Neurol* 21(3):619-21.

Folstein S, Rutter M. 1977. Infantile autism: a genetic study of 21 twin pairs. *J Child Psychol Psychiatry* 18(4):297-321.

Fombonne E. 1999. The epidemiology of autism: a review. *Psychol Med* 29(4):769-86.

Fombonne E. 2001a. Is there an epidemic of autism? *Pediatrics* 411-13.

Fombonne E. 2001b. Presentation to Immunization Safety Review Committee. *Epidemiological Slide Set.* Washington, DC.

Fombonne E. 2001c. Presentation to Immunization Safety Review Committee. *New Studies.* Washington, DC.

Fombonne E. 2002. Epidemiological trends in rates of autism. *Mol Psychiatry* 7 (Suppl 2):S4-6.

Fombonne E. 2003. The prevalence of autism. *JAMA* 289(1):87-9.

Fombonne E, Chakrabarti S. 2001. No evidence for a new variant of measles-mumps-rubella-induced autism. *Pediatrics* 108(4):E58.

Geier DA, Geier MR. 2003a. An assessment of the impact of thimerosal on childhood neurodevelopmental disorders. *Pediatr Rehabil* 6(2):97-102.

Geier M, Geier D. 2003b. Neurodevelopmental disorders after thimerosal-containing vaccines: a brief communication. *Exp Biol Med (Maywood)* 228(6):660-4.

Geier M, Geier D. 2003c. Pediatric MMR vaccination safety. *Int Pediatrics* 18(2):203-8.

Geier MR, Geier DA. 2003d. Thimerosal in childhood vaccines, neurodevelopmental disorders, and heart disease in the United States. *J Amer Phys Sur* 8(1):6-11.

Geier DA, Geier MR. 2004a. A comparative evaluation of the effects of MMR immunization and mercury doses from thimerosal-containing childhood vaccines on the population prevalence of autism. *Med Sci Monit* 10(3):PI33-9.

Geier D, Geier M. 2004b. Presentation to the Immunization Safety Review Committee. *From Epidemiology, Clinical Medicine, Molecular Biology, and Atoms, to Politics: A Review of the Relationship between Thimerosal and Autism.* Washington, DC.

Geier D, Geier M. 2004c. Submission to the Immunization Safety Review Committee. *From Epidemiology, Clinical Medicine, Molecular Biology, and Atoms, to Politics: A Review of the Relationship Between Thimerosal and Autism.*

General Biologics Product Standards. 2000. Constituent materials. *21 CFR.*610.15.

Gillberg C, Heijbel H. 1998. MMR and autism. *Autism* 2:423-4.

Gillberg C, Wing L. 1999. Autism: not an extremely rare disorder. *Acta Psychiatr Scand* 99(6):399-406.

Gillberg C, Steffenburg S, Schaumann H. 1991. Is autism more common now than ten years ago? *British J Psychiatry* 158:403-9.

Greenberg M, Pellitteri O, Barton J. 1957. Frequency of defects in infants whose mothers had rubella during pregnancy. *J Am Med Assoc* 165(6):675-8.

Gupta S, Aggarwal S, Heads C. 1996. Dysregulated immune system in children with autism: beneficial effects of intravenous immune globulin on autistic characteristics. *J Autism Dev Disord* 26(4):439-52.

Gupta S, Aggarwal S, Rashanravan B, Lee T. 1998. Th1- and Th2-like cytokines in CD4+ and CD8+ T cells in autism. *J Neuroimmunol* 85(1):106-9.

Gurney JG, Fritz MS, Ness KK, Sievers P, Newschaffer CJ, Shapiro EG. 2003. Analysis of prevalence trends of autism spectrum disorder in Minnesota. *Arch Pediatr Adolesc Med* 157(7):622-7.

Halsey NA, Goldman L. 2001. Balancing risks and benefits: primum non nocere is too simplistic. *Pediatrics* 108(2):466-7.

Hill AB. 1965. The environment and disease: association or causation? *Proc R Soc Med.* 58:295-300.

Hinestrosa C. 2001. What is Project Lead? *(Slide Presentation- Hard Copy).*

Holmes AS, Blaxill MF, Haley BE. 2003. Reduced levels of mercury in first baby haircuts of autistic children. *Int J Toxicol* 22:277-85.

Hornig M. 2004. Presentation to the Immunization Safety Review Committee. *Etiologic Factors and Pathogenesis of Autism: Evidence from Clinical Studies and Animal Models.* Washington, DC.

Hornig M, Weissenbock H, Horscroft N, Lipkin WI. 1999. An infection-based model of neurodevelopmental damage. *Proc Natl Acad Sci USA* 96(21):12102-7.

Hoshino Y, Kaneko M, Yashima Y, Kumashiro H, Volkmar FR, Cohen DJ. 1987. Clinical features of autistic children with setback course in their infancy. *Jpn J Psychiatry Neurol* 41(2):237-45.

Hviid A, Stellfeld M, Wohlfahrt J, Melbye M. 2003. Association between thimerosal-containing vaccine and autism. *JAMA* 290(13):1763-6.

Ingram JL, Stodgell CJ, Hyman SL, Figlewicz DA, Weitkamp LR, Rodier PM. 2000. Discovery of allelic variants of HOXA1 and HOXB1: genetic susceptibility to autism spectrum disorders [In Process Citation]. *Teratology* 62(6):393-405.

IOM (Institute of Medicine). 1991. *Adverse Events Following Pertussis and Rubella Vaccines.* Washington, DC: National Academy Press.

IOM. 1994a. *Adverse Events Associated with Childhood Vaccines: Evidence Bearing on Causality.* Washington, DC: National Academy Press.

IOM. 1994b. *DPT Vaccine and Chronic Nervous System Dysfunction: A New Analysis.* Washington, DC: National Academy Press.

IOM. 2001a. *Immunization Safety Review: Measles-Mumps-Rubella Vaccine and Autism.* Washington, DC: National Academy Press.

IOM. 2001b. *Immunization Safety Review: Thimerosal-Containing Vaccines and Neurodevelopmental Disorders.* Washington, DC: National Academy Press

IOM. 2002a. *Immunization Safety Review: Hepatitis B Vaccine and Demyelinating Neurological Disorders.* Washington, DC: National Academy Press.

IOM. 2002b. *Immunization Safety Review: Multiple Immunizations and Immune Dysfunction.* Washington, DC: National Academy Press.

IOM. 2002c. *Immunization Safety Review: SV40 Contamination of Polio Vaccine and Cancer.* Washington, DC: National Academies Press.

IOM. 2003. *Immunization Safety Review: Sudden Unexpected Death in Infancy.* Washington, DC: National Academies Press.

IOM. 2004. *Immunization Safety Review: Influenza Vaccines and Neurological Complications.* Washington, DC: National Academies Press.

James J. 2004. Impaired transsulfuration and oxidative stress in autistic children: Improvement with targeted nutritional intervention. Submitted to the Immunization Safety Review Committee by Bradstreet J.

Jyonouchi H, Sun S, Le H. 2001. Proinflammatory and regulatory cytokine production associated with innate and adaptive immune responses in children with autism spectrum disorders and developmental regression. *J Neuroimmunol* 120(1-2):170-9.

Kaye JA, del Mar Melero-Montes M, Jick H. 2001. Mumps, measles, and rubella vaccine and the incidence of autism recorded by general practitioners: a time trend analysis. *British Med J.* 322(7284):460-3.

Kielinen M, Rantala H, Timonen E, Linna SL, Moilanen I. 2004. Associated medical disorders and disabilities in children with autistic disorder: a population-based study. *Autism* 8(1):49-60.

Kleinbaum DG, Kupper LL, Morgenstern H. 1982. *Epidemiologic Research: Principles and Quantitative Methods.* Belmont, CA: Lifetime Learning Publications, Wadsworth, Inc.

Korvatska E, Van de Water J, Anders TF, Gershwin ME. 2002. Genetic and immunologic considerations in autism. *Neurobiol Dis* 9(2):107-25.

Krause I, He XS, Gershwin ME, Shoenfeld Y. 2002. Brief report: immune factors in autism: a critical review. *J Autism Dev Disord* 32 (4):337-45.

Kurita H. 1985. Infantile autism with speech loss before the age of thirty months. *J Am Acad Child Psychiatry* 24(2):191-6.

Last JM, Abramson JH, Friedman GD, Porta M, Spasoff RA, Thuriaux M. 1995. *A Dictionary of Epidemiology.* 3rd ed. New York: Oxford University Press.

Lord C. 1995. Follow-up of two-year-olds referred for possible autism. *J Child Psychol Psychiatry* 36(8):1365-82.

Madsen KM, Hviid A, Vestergaard M, Schendel D, Wohlfahrt J, Thorsen P, Olsen J, Melbye M. 2002. A population-based study of measles, mumps, and rubella vaccination and autism. *N Engl J Med* 347(19):1477-82.

Madsen KM, Lauritsen MB, Pedersen CB, Thorsen P, Plesner AM, Andersen PH, Mortensen PB. 2003. Thimerosal and the occurrence of autism: negative ecological evidence from Danish population-based data. *Pediatrics* 112(3 Pt 1):604-6.

Maestro S, Muratori F, Cavallaro MC, Pei F, Stern D, Golse B, Palacio-Espasa F. 2002. Attentional skills during the first 6 months of age in autism spectrum disorder. *J Am Acad Child Adolesc Psychiatry* 41(10):1239-45.

Mahaffey KR, Clickner RP, Bodurow CC. 2004. Blood organic mercury and dietary mercury intake: national health and nutrition examination survey, 1999 and 2000. *Environ Health Perspect* 112(5):562-70.

Makani S, Gollapudi S, Yel L, Chiplunkar S, Gupta S. 2002. Biochemical and molecular basis of thimerosal-induced apoptosis in T cells: a major role of mitochondrial pathway. *Genes Immun* 3(5):270-8.

Makela A, Nuorti JP, Peltola H. 2002. Neurologic disorders after measles-mumps-rubella vaccination. *Pediatrics* 110(5):957-63.

Mann J. 2003. Questions about thimerosal remain. *Exp Biol Med* 228(9):991-2; discussion 993-4.

Mars AE, Mauk JE, Dowrick PW. 1998. Symptoms of pervasive developmental disorders as observed in prediagnostic home videos of infants and toddlers. *J Pediatr* 132(3 Pt 1):500-4.

Micali N, Chakrabarti S, Fombonne E. 2004. The broad autism phenotype: findings from an epidemiological survey. *Autism* 8(1):21-37.

Miller E. 2004. Presentation to the Immunization Safety Review Committee. *Thimerosal and Developmental Problems Including Autism.* Washington, DC.

Moore SJ, Turnpenny P, Quinn A, Glover S, Lloyd DJ, Montgomery T, Dean JC. 2000. A clinical study of 57 children with fetal anticonvulsant syndromes. *J Med Genet* 37(7):489-97.

Mullooly J, Drew L, DeStefano F, Chen R, Okoro K, Swint E, Immanuel V, Ray P, Lewis N, Vadheim C, Lugg M. 1999. Quality of HMO vaccination databases used to monitor childhood vaccine safety. *Am J Epidemiol* 149(2):186-94.

Murch SH, Anthony A, Casson D, Malik M, Berelowitz M, Dhillon AP, Thomson MA, Valentine A, Davies SE, Walker-Smith JA. 2004. Retraction of an Interpretation. *Lancet* 363:750.

Nan X, Ng HH, Johnson CA, Laherty CD, Turner BM, Eisenman RN, Bird A. 1998. Transcriptional repression by the methyl-CpG-binding protein MeCP2 involves a histone deacetylase complex. *Nature* 393(6683):386-9.

Nelson KB, Bauman ML. 2003. Thimerosal and autism? *Pediatrics* 111(3):674-9.

Nelson KB, Grether JK, Croen LA, Dambrosia JM, Dickens BF, Jelliffe LL, Hansen RL, Phillips TM. 2001. Neuropeptides and neurotrophins in neonatal blood of children with autism or mental retardation. *Ann Neurol* 49(5):597-606.

Nordin J. 2004. Commentary on data presented by the Geiers at the Thimerosal meeting. Email to Immunization Safety Review Committee (imsafety@nas.edu). March 11.

NRC (National Research Council). 1989. *Improving Risk Communication.* Washington, DC: National Academy Press.

NRC. 2000. *Toxicological Effects of Methylmercury.* Washington, DC: National Academy Press.

Osterling J, Dawson G. 1994. Early recognition of children with autism: a study of first birthday home videotapes. *J Autism Dev Disord* 24(3):247-57.

Patja A, Davidkin I, Kurki T, Kallio MJ, Valle M, Peltola H. 2000. Serious adverse events after measles-mumps-rubella vaccination during a fourteen-year prospective follow-up. [In Process Citation]. *Pediatr Infect Dis J* 19(12):1127-34.

Pavone P, Bianchini R, Parano E, Incorpora G, Rizzo R, Mazzone L, Trifiletti RR. 2004. Anti-brain antibodies in PANDAS versus uncomplicated streptococcal infection. *Pediatr Neurol* 30(2):107-10.

Peltola H, Patja A, Leinikki P, Valle M, Davidkin I, Paunio M. 1998. No evidence for measles, mumps, and rubella vaccine-associated inflammatory bowel disease or autism in a 14-year prospective study [letter]. *Lancet* 351(9112):1327-8.

Persico AM, D'Agruma L, Maiorano N, Totaro A, Militerni R, Bravaccio C, Wassink TH, Schneider C, Melmed R, Trillo S, Montecchi F, Palermo M, Pascucci T, Puglisi-Allegra S, Reichelt KL, Conciatori M, Marino R, Quattrocchi CC, Baldi A, Zelante L, Gasparini P, Keller F. 2001. Reelin gene alleles and haplotypes as a factor predisposing to autistic disorder. *Mol Psychiatry* 6(2):150-9.

Pichichero ME, Cernichiari E, Lopreiato J, Treanor J. 2002. Mercury concentrations and metabolism in infants receiving vaccines containing thiomersal: a descriptive study. *Lancet* 360(9347):1737-41.

Plioplys AV. 2000. Intravenous immunoglobulin treatment in autism. *J Autism Dev Disord* 30(1):73-4.

Rapin I. 1997. Autism. *New Engl J Med* 337(2):97-104.

Ritvo ER, Freeman BJ, Pingree C, Mason-Brothers A, Jorde L, Jenson WR, McMahon WM, Petersen PB, Mo A, Ritvo A. 1989a. The UCLA-University of Utah epidemiologic survey of autism: prevalence. *Am J Psychiatry* 146(2):194-9.

Ritvo ER, Jorde LB, Mason-Brothers A, Freeman BJ, Pingree C, Jones MB, McMahon WM, Petersen PB, Jenson WR, Mo A. 1989b. The UCLA-University of Utah epidemiologic survey of autism: recurrence risk estimates and genetic counseling. *Am J Psychiatry* 146(8):1032-6.

Rogan WJ, Dietrich KN, Ware JH, Dockery DW, Salganik M, Radcliffe J, Jones RL, Ragan NB, Chisolm JJ Jr, Rhoads GG. 2001. The effect of chelation therapy with succimer on neuropsychological development in children exposed to lead. *N Engl J Med* 344(19):1421-6.

Rogers SJ, DiLalla DL. 1990. Age of symptom onset in young children with pervasive developmental disorders. *J Am Acad Child Adolesc Psychiatry* 29(6):863-72.

Rosenthal S, Chen R, Hadler S. 1996. The safety of acellular pertussis vaccine vs whole-cell pertussis vaccine. A postmarketing assessment. *Arch Pediatr Adolesc Med* 150(5):457-60.

Rumsey JM, Ernst M. 2000. Functional neuroimaging of autistic disorders. *Ment Retard Dev Disabil Res Rev* 6(3):171-9.

Rutter M. 1999. The Emanuel Miller Memorial Lecture 1998. Autism: two-way interplay between research and clinical work. *J Child Psychol Psychiatry* 40(2):169-88.

SafeMinds. 2000. VSD subgroup analysis of Spring 2000: Background information on this document. Submitted by S. Bernard on Behalf of SafeMinds. January 18.

SafeMinds. 2003. Analysis and critique of the CDC's handling of the thimerosal exposure assessment based on Vaccine Safety Datalink (VSD) information. Submitted by S. Bernard on Behalf of SafeMinds. January 18:1-46.

SafeMinds. 2004a. VSD thimerosal analysis of 2/29/00: Background information on this document. Submitted by S. Bernard on Behalf of SafeMinds. January 18.

SafeMinds. 2004b. VSD thimerosal analysis of June 2000: Background information on this document. Submitted by S. Bernard on Behalf of SafeMinds. January 18.

SafeMinds. 2004c. VSD Thimerosal Study Protocol: Background information on this document. Submitted by S. Bernard on Behalf of SafeMinds. January 18.

Sager P. 2004. Presentation to the Immunization Safety Review Committee. *NIAID Studies on Thimerosal*. Washington, DC.

Salisbury D. 2004. Autism and vaccines. E-mail to Stratton K. January 29, 2004. *Attachment: transcript of a High Court hearing in the United Kingdom.*

Sandborgh Englund G, Dahlqvist R, Lindelof B, Soderman E, Jonzon B, Vesterberg O, Larsson KS. 1994. DMSA administration to patients with alleged mercury poisoning from dental amalgams: A placebo-controlled study. *J Dent Res* 73(3):620-28.

Schober SE, Sinks TH, Jones RL, Bolger PM, McDowell M, Osterloh J, Garrett ES, Canady RA, Dillon CF, Sun Y, Joseph CB, Mahaffey KR. 2003. Blood mercury levels in US children and women of childbearing age, 1999-2000. *JAMA* 289(13):1667-74.

Sheils O, Smyth P, Martin C, O'Leary JJ. 2002. Development of an 'allelic discrimination' type assay to differentiate between the strain origens of measles virus detected in intestinal tissue of children with ileocolonic lymphonodular hyperplasia and concomitant developmental disorder. *J Virol* 75(2):910-20.

Simpsonwood Retreat Center. 2000. Transcript. Scientific Review of Vaccine Safety Datalink Information, June 7-8. Norcross, GA: Simpsonwood Retreat Center.

Singh VK. 1996. Plasma increase of interleukin-12 and interferon-gamma. Pathological significance in autism. *J Neuroimmunol* 66(1-2):143-5.

Singh VK. 2004. Submission to the Immunization Safety Review. *Autism, Vaccines, and Immune Reactions.* Washington, DC.

Singh VK, Fudenberg HH, Emerson D, Coleman M. 1988. Immunodiagnosis and immunotherapy in autistic children. *Ann NY Acad Sci* 540:602-4.

Singh VK, Warren RP, Odell JD, Cole P. 1991. Changes of soluble interleukin-2, interleukin-2 receptor, T8 antigen, and interleukin-1 in the serum of autistic children. *Clin Immunol Immunopathol* 61(3):448-55.

Singh VK, Warren RP, Odell JD, Warren WL, Cole P. 1993. Antibodies to myelin basic protein in children with autistic behavior. *Brain Behav Immun* 7(1):97-103.

Singh VK, Warren R, Averett R, Ghaziuddin M. 1997. Circulating autoantibodies to neuronal and glial filament proteins in autism. *Pediatr Neurol* 17(1):88-90.

Singleton JA, Lloyd JC, Mootrey GT, Salive ME, Chen RT. 1999. An overview of the vaccine adverse event reporting system (VAERS) as a surveillance system. *Vaccine* 17:2908-17.

Slovic P. 1999. Trust, emotion, sex, politics, and science: surveying the risk-assessment battlefield. *Risk Anal* 19(4):689-701.

Smith CM, Wang X, Hu H, Kelsey KT. 1995. A polymorphism in the delta-aminolevulinic acid dehydratase gene may modify the pharmacokinetics and toxicity of lead. *Environ Health Perspect* 103(3):248-53.

Steffenburg S, Gillberg C, Hellgren L, Andersson L, Gillberg IC, Jakobsson G, Bohman M. 1989. A twin study of autism in Denmark, Finland, Iceland, Norway and Sweden. *J Child Psychol Psychiatry* 30(3):405-16.

Stehr-Green P, Tull P, Stellfeld M, Mortenson PB, Simpson D. 2003. Autism and thimerosal-containing vaccines: lack of consistent evidence for an association. *Am J Prev Med* 25(2):101-6.

Stromland K, Nordin V, Miller M, Akerstrom B, Gillberg C. 1994. Autism in thalidomide embryopathy: a population study. *Dev Med Child Neurol* 36(4):351-6.

Stubbs EG, Crawford ML. 1977. Depressed lymphocyte responsiveness in autistic children. *J Autism Child Schizophr* 7(1):49-55.

Swedo SE, Leonard HL, Garvey M, Mittleman B, Allen AJ, Perlmutter S, Lougee L, Dow S, Zamkoff J, Dubbert BK. 1998. Pediatric autoimmune neuropsychiatric disorders associated with streptococcal infections: clinical description of the first 50 cases. *Am J Psychiatry* 155(2):264-71.

Sweeten TL, Bowyer SL, Posey DJ, Halberstadt GM, McDougle CJ. 2003. Increased prevalence of familial autoimmunity in probands with pervasive developmental disorders. *Pediatrics* 112(5):e420-4.

Takahashi H, Suzumura S, Shirakizawa F, Wada N, Tanaka-Taya K, Arai S, Okabe N, Ichikawa H, Sato T. 2003. An epidemiological study on Japanese autism concerning routine childhood immunization history. *Jpn J Infect Dis* 56(3):114-7.

Taylor B, Miller E, Farrington CP. 2000. Response to the MMR question. *Lancet* 7;356(9237):1273.

Taylor B, Miller E, Farrington CP, Petropoulos MC, Favot-Mayaud I, Li J, Waight PA. 1999. Autism and measles, mumps, and rubella vaccine: No epidemiological evidence for a causal association. *Lancet* 353(9169):2026-9.

Taylor B, Miller E, Lingam R, Andrews N, Simmons ASJ. 2002. Measles, mumps, and rubella vaccination and bowel problems or developmental regression in children with autism: population study. *British Med J* 324(7334):393-6.

Todd RD, Ciaranello RD. 1985. Demonstration of inter- and intraspecies differences in serotonin binding sites by antibodies from an autistic child. *Proc Natl Acad Sci USA* 82(2):612-6.

Torrente F, Ashwood P, Day R, Machado N, Furlano RI, Anthony A, Davies SE, Wakefield AJ, Thomson MA, Walker-Smith JA, Murch SH. 2002. Small intestinal enteropathy with epithelial IgG and complement deposition in children with regressive autism. *Mol Psychiatry* 7(4):375-82, 334.

Trottier G, Srivastava L, Walker CD. 1999. Etiology of infantile autism: a review of recent advances in genetic and neurobiological research. *J Psychiatry Neurosci* 24(2):103-15.

Tuchman RF, Rapin I. 1997. Regression in pervasive developmental disorders: seizures and epileptiform electroencephalogram correlates. *Pediatrics* 99(4):560-6.

Tuchman RF, Rapin I, Shinnar S. 1991. Autistic and dysphasic children. I: Clinical characteristics. *Pediatrics* 88(6):1211-8.

Uhlmann V, Martin CM, Sheils O, Pilkington L, Silva I, Killalea A, Murch SB, Wakefield AJ, O'Leary JJ. 2002. Potential viral pathogenic mechanism for new variant inflammatory bowel disease. *J Clin Pathol: Mol Pathol.* 55(2):84-90.

Varricchio F. 1998. The vaccine adverse event reporting system. *J Toxicol Clin Toxicol* 36(7):765-8.

Varricchio F, Iskander J, Destefano F, Ball R, Pless R, Braun MM, Chen RT. 2004. Understanding vaccine safety information from the Vaccine Adverse Event Reporting System. *J Pediatr Infect Dis* 23(4):287-94.

Verstraeten T. 2001. Presentation to Immunization Safety Review Committee. *Vaccine Safety Datalink (VSD) Screening Study and Follow-Up Analysis with Harvard Pilgrim Data.* Washington, DC.

Verstraeten T. 2004. Thimerosal, the Centers for Disease Control and Prevention, and GlaxoSmithKline. *Pediatrics* 113(4):932.

Verstraeten T, Davis RL, DeStefano F, Lieu TA, Rhodes PH, Black SB, Shinefield H, Chen RT, Vaccine Safety Datalink Team. 2003. Safety of thimerosal-containing vaccines: a two-phased study of computerized health maintenance organization databases. *Pediatrics* 112(5):1039-48.

Vojdani A, Campbell AW, Anyanwu E, Kashanian A, Bock K, Vojdani E. 2002. Antibodies to neuron-specific antigens in children with autism: possible cross-reaction with encephalitogenic proteins from milk, Chlamydia pneumoniae and Streptococcus group A. *J Neuroimmunol* 129(1-2):168-77.

Volkmar F. 2001. Presentation to Immunization Safety Review Committee. *Diagnosis of Autism.* Washington, DC.

Volkmar F, Pauls D. 2003. Autism. *Lancet* 362:1133-41.

Wakefield AJ, Murch SH, Anthony A, Linnell J, Casson DM, Malik M, Berelowitz M, Dhillon AP, Thomson MA, Harvey P, Valentine A, Davies SE, Walker-Smith JA. 1998. Ileal-lymphoid-nodular hyperplasia, non-specific colitis, and pervasive developmental disorder in children. *Lancet* 351(9103):637-41.

Wakefield AJ, Anthony A, Murch SH, Thomson M, Montgomery SM, Davies S, O'Leary JJ, Berelowitz M, Walker-Smith JA. 2000. Enterocolitis in children with developmental disorders [see comments]. *Am J Gastroenterol* 95(9):2285-95.

Wakefield AJ, Puleston JM, Montgomery SM, Anthony A, O'Leary JJ, Murch SH. 2002. Review article: the concept of entero-colonic encephalopathy, autism and opioid receptor ligands. *Aliment Pharmacol Ther* 16(4):663-74.

Walsh W, Usman A. 2001. Metallothionein Dysfunction in Children Diagnosed with Autism Spectrum Disorders. Poster: American Psychiatric Accosciation Annual Meeting, May 10, 2001. Pfeiffer Treatment Center, IL.

Waly M, Olteanu H, Banerjee R, Choi SW, Mason JB, Parker BS, Sukumar S, Shim S, Sharma A, Benzecry JM, Power-Charnitsky VA, Deth RC. 2004. Activation of methionine synthase by insulin-like growth factor-1 and dopamine: a target for neurodevelopmental toxins and thimerosal. *Mol Psychiatry* 9(4):358-70.

Warren Grant Magnuson Clinical Center, National Institutes of Health. 2004. Preparing for Transfusion Therapy. Online: http://www.healthfinder.gov/orgs/HR0022.htm.

Warren RP, Margaretten NC, Pace NC, Foster A. 1986. Immune abnormalities in patients with autism. *J Autism Dev Disord* 16(2):189-97.

Warren RP, Foster A, Margaretten NC. 1987. Reduced natural killer cell activity in autism. *J Am Acad Child Adolesc Psychiatry* 26(3):333-5.

Warren RP, Singh VK, Cole P, Odell JD, Pingree CB, Warren WL, White E. 1991. Increased frequency of the null allele at the complement C4b locus in autism. *Clin Exp Immunol* 83(3):438-40.

Warren RP, Singh VK, Cole P, Odell JD, Pingree CB, Warren WL, DeWitt CW, McCullough M. 1992. Possible association of the extended MHC haplotype B44-SC30-DR4 with autism. *Immunogenetics* 36(4):203-7.

Warren RP, Odell JD, Warren WL, Burger RA, Maciulis A, Daniels WW, Torres AR. 1996. Strong association of the third hypervariable region of HLA-DR beta 1 with autism. *J Neuroimmunol* 67(2):97-102.

Wassink TH, Piven J, Vieland VJ, Huang J, Swiderski RE, Pietila J, Braun T, Beck G, Folstein SE, Haines JL, Sheffield VC. 2001. Evidence supporting WNT2 as an autism susceptibility gene. *Am J Med Genet* 105(5):406-13.

Watson JC, Redd SC, Rhodes PH, Hadler SC. 1998. The interruption of transmission of indigenous measles in the United States during 1993. *Pediatr Infect Dis J* 17(5):363-6; discussion 366-7.

Weed DL, Hursting SD. 1998. Biologic plausibility in causal inference: current method and practice. *Am J Epidemiol* 147(5):415-25.

Wentz P.W. 2000. Chelation therapy: conventional treatments. *Advance/Laboratory*. Available at http://www.advanceforAL.com.

Werner E, Dawson G, Munson J, Osterling J. In Press. Variation in early developmental course in autism and its relation with behavioral outcome at 3-4 years of age. *J Autism Dev Disorder*.

Wilson GS. 1967. *The Hazards of Immunization.* New York: The Athlone Press. Pp. 75-84.

Wilson K. 2004. Presentation to the Immunization Safety Review Committee. Washington, DC.

Wilson K, Mills E, Ross C, McGowan J, Jadad A. 2003. Association of autistic spectrum disorder and the measles, mumps, and rubella vaccine: a systematic review of current epidemiological evidence. *Arch Pediatr Adolesc Med* 157(7):628-34.

Wing L, Potter D. 2002. The epidemiology of autistic spectrum disorders: is the prevalence rising? *Mental Ret Dev Disabil Res Rev* 8:151-61.

Yeargin-Allsopp M, Rice C, Karapurkar T, Doernberg N, Boyle C, Murphy C. 2003. Prevalence of autism in a US metropolitan area. *JAMA* 289(1):49-55.

Zimmerman AW. 2000. Commentary: immunological treatments for autism: in search of reasons for promising approaches. *J Autism Dev Disord* 30(5):481-4.

Zoghbi HY. 2003. Postnatal neurodevelopmental disorders: meeting at the synapse? *Science* 302(5646):826-30.

Appendix A

Committee Recommendations and Conclusions from Previous Reports

MEASLES-MUMPS-RUBELLA VACCINE AND AUTISM

Conclusions

The committee concludes that the evidence favors rejection of a causal relationship at the population level between measles-mumps-rubella (MMR) vaccine and autistic spectrum disorders (ASD). However, this conclusion does not exclude the possibility that MMR vaccine could contribute to ASD in a small number of children.

The committee concludes that further research on the possible occurrence of ASD in a small number of children subsequent to MMR vaccination is warranted, and it has identified targeted research opportunities that could lead to firmer understanding of the relationship.

Recommendations

Public Health Response

The committee recommends that the relationship between the MMR vaccine and autistic spectrum disorders receive continued attention.

Policy Review

The committee does not recommend a policy review at this time of the licensure of MMR vaccine or of the current schedule and recommendations for administration of MMR vaccine.

Research Regarding MMR and ASD

The committee recommends the use of accepted and consistent case definitions and assessment protocols for ASD in order to enhance the precision and comparability of results from surveillance, epidemiological, and biological investigations.

The committee recommends the exploration of whether exposure to MMR vaccine is a risk factor for autistic spectrum disorder in a small number of children.

The committee recommends the development of targeted investigations of whether or not measles vaccine-strain virus is present in the intestines of some children with ASD.

The committee encourages all who submit reports to VAERS of any diagnosis of ASD thought to be related to MMR vaccine to provide as much detail and as much documentation as possible.

The committee recommends studying the possible effects of different MMR immunization exposures.

The committee recommends conducting further clinical and epidemiological studies of sufficient rigor to identify risk factors and biological markers of ASD in order to better understand genetic or environmental causes.

Communications

The committee recommends that government agencies and professional organizations, CDC and the Food and Drug Administration (FDA) in particular, review some of the most prominent forms of communication regarding the hypothesized relationship between MMR vaccine and ASD, including information they provide via the Internet and the ease with which Internet information can be accessed.

THIMEROSAL-CONTAINING VACCINES AND NEURODEVELOPMENTAL DISORDERS

Conclusions

The committee concludes that although the hypothesis that exposure to thimerosal-containing vaccines could be associated with neurodevelopmental disorders is not established and rests on indirect and incomplete information, primarily from analogies with methylmercury and levels of maximum mercury exposure from vaccines given in children, the hypothesis is biologically plausible.

The committee also concludes that the evidence is inadequate to accept or reject a causal relationship between thimerosal exposures from childhood vaccines and the neurodevelopmental disorders of autism, ADHD, and speech or language delay.

Public Health Response Recommendations

Policy Review and Analysis

The committee recommends the use of the thimerosal-free DTaP, Hib, and hepatitis B vaccines in the United States, despite the fact that there might be remaining supplies of thimerosal-containing vaccine available.

The committee recommends that full consideration be given by appropriate professional societies and government agencies to removing thimerosal from vaccines administered to infants, children, or pregnant women in the United States.

The committee recommends that appropriate professional societies and government agencies review their policies about the non-vaccine biological and pharmaceutical products that contain thimerosal and are used by infants, children, and pregnant women in the United States.

The committee recommends that policy analyses be conducted that will inform these discussions in the future.

The committee recommends a review and assessment of how public health policy decisions are made under uncertainty.

The committee recommends a review of the strategies used to communicate rapid changes in vaccine policy, and it recommends research on how to improve those strategies.

Public Health and Biomedical Research

The committee recommends a diverse public health and biomedical research portfolio.

Epidemiological Research

The committee recommends case-control studies examining the potential link between neurodevelopmental disorders and thimerosal-containing vaccines.

The committee recommends further analysis of neurodevelopmental disorders in cohorts of children who did not receive thimerosal-containing doses as part of a clinical trial of DTaP vaccine.

The committee recommends conducting epidemiological studies that compare the incidence and prevalence of neurodevelopmental disorders before and after the removal of thimerosal from vaccines.

The committee recommends an increased effort to identify the primary sources and levels of prenatal and postnatal background exposure to thimerosal (e.g., Rho (D) Immune Globulin) and other forms of mercury (e.g., maternal consumption of fish) in infants, children, and pregnant women.

Clinical Research

The committee recommends research on how children, including those diagnosed with neurodevelopmental disorders, metabolize and excrete metals—particularly mercury.

The committee recommends continued research on theoretical modeling of ethylmercury exposures, including the incremental burden of thimerosal with background mercury exposure from other sources.

The committee recommends careful, rigorous, and scientific investigations of chelation when used in children with neurodevelopmental disorders, especially autism.

Basic Science Research

The committee recommends research to identify a safe, effective, and inexpensive alternative to thimerosal for countries that decide they need to switch from using thimerosal as a preservative.

The committee recommends research in appropriate animal models on the neurodevelopmental effects of ethylmercury.

MULTIPLE IMMUNIZATIONS AND IMMUNE DYSFUNCTION

Conclusions

Scientific Assessment

Causality Conclusions

The committee concludes that the epidemiological evidence favors rejection of a causal relationship between multiple immunizations and an increase in heterologous infection.

The committee concludes that the epidemiological evidence favors rejection of a causal relationship between multiple immunizations and an increased risk of type 1 diabetes.

The committee concludes that the epidemiological evidence is inadequate to accept or reject a causal relationship between multiple immunizations and increased risk of allergic disease, particularly asthma.

Biological Mechanisms Conclusions

Autoimmune Disease

In the absence of experimental or human evidence regarding molecular mimicry or mercury-induced modification of any vaccine component to create an antigenic epitope capable of cross-reaction with self epitopes as a mechanism by which multiple immunizations under the U.S. infant immunization schedule could possibly influence an individual's risk of autoimmunity, the committee concludes that these mechanisms are only theoretical.

The committee concludes that there is weak evidence for bystander activation, alone or in concert with molecular mimicry, as a mechanism by which multiple immunizations under the U.S. infant immunization schedule could possibly influence an individual's risk of autoimmunity.

In the absence of experimental or human evidence regarding loss of protection against a homologous infection as a mechanism by which multiple immunizations under the U.S. infant immunization schedule could possibly influence an individual's risk of autoimmunity, the committee concludes that this mechanism is only theoretical.

In the absence of experimental or human evidence regarding mechanisms related to the hygiene hypothesis as a means by which multiple immunizations under the U.S. infant immunization schedule could possibly influence an individual's risk of autoimmunity, the committee concludes that this mechanism is only theoretical.

Considering molecular mimicry, bystander activation, and impaired immunoregulation collectively rather than individually, the committee concludes that there is weak evidence for these mechanisms as means by which multiple immunizations under the U.S. infant immunization schedule could possibly influence an individual's risk of autoimmunity.

Allergic Disease

The committee concludes that there is weak evidence for bystander activation as a mechanism by which multiple immunizations under the U.S. infant immunization schedule could possibly influence an individual's risk of allergy.

In the absence of experimental or human evidence regarding mechanisms related to the hygiene hypothesis as a means by which multiple immunizations under the U.S. infant immunization schedule could possibly influence an individual's risk of allergy, the committee concludes that this mechanism is only theoretical.

The committee concludes that there is weak evidence for the existence of any biological mechanisms, collectively or individually, by which multiple immunizations under the U.S. infant immunization schedule could possibly influence an individual's risk of allergy.

Heterologous Infection

The committee concludes that there is strong evidence for the existence of biological mechanisms by which multiple immunizations under the U.S. infant immunization schedule could possibly influence an individual's risk for heterologous infections.

Significance Assessment

The committee concludes that concern about multiple immunizations has been, and could continue to be, of societal significance in terms of parental worries, potential health burdens, and future challenges for immunization policymaking.

Public Health Response Recommendations

Policy Review

The committee recommends that state and federal vaccine policymakers consider a broader and more explicit strategy for developing recommendations for the use of vaccines.

The committee does not recommend a policy review—by the CDC's Advisory Committee on Immunization Practices (ACIP), the American Academy of Pediatrics' Committee on Infectious Diseases, and the American Academy of Family Physicians—of the current recommended childhood immunization schedule on the basis of concerns about immune system dysfunction.

The committee does not recommend a policy review by the Food and Drug Administration's Vaccines and Related Biologic Products Advisory Committee of any currently licensed vaccines on the basis of concerns about immune system dysfunction.

Research

Epidemiological Research

The committee recommends exploring the feasibility of using existing vaccine surveillance systems, alone or in combination, to study safety questions related to asthma and other important allergic disorders, as well as to type 1 diabetes and other important autoimmune diseases.

The committee recommends exploring the use of cohorts for research on possible vaccine-related disease risks. Furthermore, the committee recommends that disease registries and research programs for autoimmune and allergic disorders routinely collect immunization histories as part of their study protocol.

Basic Science and Clinical Research

The committee recommends continued research on the development of the human infant immune system.

The committee endorses current research efforts aimed at identifying genetic variability in human immune system development and immune system responsiveness as a way to gain a better understanding of genetic susceptibility to vaccine-based adverse events.

The committee recommends exploring the feasibility of collecting data on surrogate markers for autoimmune and allergic disorders in the vaccine testing and licensing process.

The committee recommends exploring surrogates for allergy and autoimmunity in existing cohort studies of variations in the vaccine schedule.

Communication

The committee recommends that an appropriate panel of multidisciplinary experts be convened by the Department of Health and Human Services. It would develop a comprehensive research strategy for knowledge leading to the optimal design and evaluation of vaccine risk-benefit communication approaches.

HEPATITIS B VACCINE AND DEMYELINATING NEUROLOGICAL DISORDERS

Scientific Assessment

Causality Conclusions

The committee concludes that the evidence favors rejection of a causal relationship between hepatitis B vaccine administered to adults and incident multiple sclerosis.

The committee also concludes that the evidence favors rejection of a causal relationship between hepatitis B vaccine administered to adults and multiple sclerosis relapse.

The committee concludes that the evidence is inadequate to accept or reject a causal relationship between hepatitis B vaccine and the first episode of a central nervous system demyelinating disorder.

The committee concludes that the evidence is inadequate to accept or reject a causal relationship between hepatitis B vaccine and ADEM.

The committee concludes that the evidence is inadequate to accept or reject a causal relationship between hepatitis B vaccine and optic neuritis.

The committee concludes that the evidence is inadequate to accept or reject a causal relationship between hepatitis B vaccine and transverse myelitis.

The committee concludes that the evidence is inadequate to accept or reject a causal relationship between hepatitis B vaccine and GBS.

The committee concludes that the evidence is inadequate to accept or reject a causal relationship between hepatitis B vaccine and brachial neuritis.

The committee concludes that there is weak evidence for biological mechanisms by which hepatitis B vaccination could possibly influence an individual's risk of the central or peripheral nervous system disorders of MS, first episode of CDD, ADEM, or optic neuritis, transverse myelitis, GBS, or brachial neuritis.

Significance Assessment

The committee concludes that concerns about the hepatitis B vaccine remain significant in the minds of some parents and workers who are required to take the vaccine because of occupational risk.

Public Health Response Recommendations

Policy Review

The committee does not recommend a policy review of the hepatitis B vaccine by any of the national and federal vaccine advisory bodies on the basis of concerns about demyelinating neurological disorders.

The committee recommends continued surveillance of hepatitis B disease and increased surveillance of secondary diseases such as cirrhosis and hepatocellular carcinoma.

Basic and Clinical Science

The committee recommends continued research in animal and *in vitro* models, as well as in humans, on the mechanisms of immune-mediated neurological disease possibly associated with exposure to vaccines.

Communication

The committee again recommends that government agencies and professional organizations responsible for immunizations critically evaluate their communication services with increased understanding of, and input from, the intended user.

SV40 CONTAMINATION OF POLIO VACCINE AND CANCER

Scientific Assessment

Causality Conclusions

The committee concludes that the evidence is inadequate to accept or reject a causal relationship between SV40-containing polio vaccines and cancer.

Biological Mechanisms Conclusions

The committee concludes that the biological evidence is strong that SV40 is a transforming virus.

The committee concludes that the biological evidence is moderate that SV40 exposure could lead to cancer in humans under natural conditions.

The committee concludes that the biological evidence is moderate that SV40 exposure from the polio vaccine is related to SV40 infection in humans.

Significance Assessment

The committee concludes that concerns about exposure to SV40 through inadvertent contamination of polio vaccines are significant because of the seriousness of cancers as the possible adverse health outcomes and because of the continuing need to ensure and protect public trust in the nation's immunization program.

Public Health Response Recommendations

Policy Review

The committee does not recommend a policy review of polio vaccine by any of the national or federal vaccine advisory bodies, on the basis of concerns about cancer risks that might be associated with exposure to SV40, because the vaccine in current use is free of SV40.

Policy Analysis and Communication

The committee recommends that the appropriate federal agencies develop a Vaccine Contamination Prevention and Response Plan.

Research

The committee recommends development of sensitive and specific serologic tests for SV40.

The committee recommends the development and use of sensitive and specific standardized techniques for SV40 detection.

The committee recommends that once there is agreement in the scientific community as to the best detection methods and protocols, pre-1955 samples of human tissues should be assayed for presence or absence of SV40 in rigorous, multi-center studies.

The committee recommends further study of the transmissibility of SV40 in humans.

Until some of the technical issues are resolved, the committee does not recommend additional epidemiological studies of people potentially exposed to the contaminated polio vaccine.

VACCINATIONS AND SUDDEN UNEXPECTED DEATH IN INFANCY

Scientific Assessment

Causality Conclusions

There is no basis for a change in the prior conclusions that the evidence favors rejection of a causal relationship between DTwP vaccine and SIDS.

The evidence is inadequate to accept or reject a causal relationship between DTaP vaccine and SIDS.

The evidence is inadequate to accept or reject causal relationships between SIDS and the individual vaccines, Hib, HepB, OPV, and IPV.

The evidence favors rejection of a causal relationship between exposure to multiple vaccines and SIDS.

The evidence is inadequate to accept or reject a causal relationship between exposure to multiple vaccines and sudden unexpected death in infancy, other than SIDS.

The evidence favors acceptance of a causal relationship between diphtheria toxoid-and whole cell pertussis vaccine and death due to anaphylaxis in infants.

The evidence is inadequate to accept or reject a causal relationship between hepatitis B vaccine and neonatal death.

Biological Mechanisms Conclusions

In the absence of experimental or human evidence regarding the ability of common side effects of immunization, including fever and anorexia, to trigger sudden unexpected death in infants with underlying neuroregulatory abnormalities, the committee concludes that this mechanisms is only theoretical.

In the absence of experimental or human evidence regarding the ability of common side effects of immunization, including fever and anorexia, to trigger an acute metabolic crisis in patients with inborn errors of metabolism, the committee concludes that this mechanism for vaccine-related sudden unexpected infant death is only theoretical.

In the absence of experimental or human evidence demonstrating the ability of vaccines to stimulate an abnormal inflammatory response in the lung leading to sudden unexpected infant death, the committee concludes that this mechanism is only theoretical.

The committee concludes that immediate type I hypersensitivity reactions to vaccines can cause SUDI within 24 hours of vaccine administration. Although a type I hypersensitivity reaction leading to death could possibly be missed both clinically and at post-mortem examination, and therefore misdiagnosed as SIDS, the committee concludes that this possibility is only theoretical.

Public Health Response Recommendations

Policy Review

The committee does not recommend a policy review of the recommended childhood vaccination schedule by any of the national or federal vaccine advisory bodies on the basis of concerns about sudden unexpected death in infancy.

Surveillance and Epidemiological Studies

The committee urges prompt publication of all Vaccine Safety Datalink results.

Basic and Clinical Science

The committee recommends continued research on the etiology and pathology of SIDS.

The committee recommends that a comprehensive postmortem workup, including a metabolic analysis, be done on all infants who die suddenly and unexpectedly.

The committee encourages efforts by Centers for Disease Control and Prevention, American Academy of Pediatrics, and others to promote the development and consistent use throughout the United States of national guidelines for investigation, diagnosis, and reporting of SIDS cases.

The committee recommends the development of standard definitions and guidance for diagnosis and reporting of SUDI for research purposes.

INFLUENZA VACCINES AND NEUROLOGICAL COMPLICATIONS

Scientific Assessment

Causality Conclusions

The committee concludes that the evidence favors acceptance of a causal relationship between 1976 swine influenza vaccine and Guillain-Barré syndrome in adults.

The committee concludes that the evidence is inadequate to accept or reject a causal relationship between GBS in adults and influenza vaccines administered after 1976 (that is, subsequent to the swine influenza vaccine program).

The committee concludes that the evidence favors rejection of a causal relationship between influenza vaccines and relapse of multiple sclerosis in adults.

The committee concludes that the evidence is inadequate to accept or reject a causal relationship between influenza vaccines and incident MS in adults.

The committee concludes that the evidence is inadequate to accept or reject a causal relationship between influenza vaccines and optic neuritis in adults.

The committee concludes that the evidence is inadequate to accept or reject a causal relationship between influenza vaccines and other demyelinating neurological disorders.

The committee concludes that there is no evidence bearing on a causal relationship between influenza vaccines and demyelinating neurological disorders in children aged 6-23 months.

Biological Mechanisms Conclusions

The committee concludes that there is weak evidence for biological mechanisms related to immune-mediated processes, including molecular mimicry and bystander activation, by which receipt of any influenza vaccine could possibly influence an individual's risk of developing the neurological complications of GBS, MS, or other demyelinating conditions such as optic neuritis.

In the absence of experimental or human evidence regarding the direct neurotoxic effect of influenza vaccines, the committee concludes that this mechanism is only theoretical.

Public Health Response Recommendations

Policy Review

The committee does not recommend a policy review of the recommendations for influenza vaccination by any of the national or federal vaccine advisory bodies on the basis of concerns about neurological complications. Current and future immunization policies should continue to reflect the benefits of influenza vaccination.

Research

The committee recommends increased surveillance of adverse events associated with influenza vaccination of children, with particular attentiveness to detecting and assessing potential neurological complications. Enhanced surveillance should be in place before an ACIP recommendation is implemented for universal annual influenza vaccination of young children.

The committee recommends efforts to develop techniques for the detection and evaluation of rare adverse events and encourages the use of administrative databases and the standardization of immunization records as part of this effort.

Basic Science and Clinical Research

The committee supports ongoing research aimed at better understanding the pathogenesis of influenza and encourages efforts to anticipate which strains might be more neurologically active.

Although stocks of the 1976 vaccine are unlikely available, the committee recommends that if samples of the influenza vaccines used in 1976 are available, they should be analyzed for the presence of *C. jejuni* antigens, NS1 or NS2 proteins, or other possible contaminants. The 1976 vaccines should be compared with current and other historical influenza vaccines.

The committee recommends continued research using animal and *in vitro* models, as well as with humans, on the mechanisms of immune-mediated neurological diseases that might be associated with exposure to vaccines.

The committee recommends continued research efforts aimed at identifying genetic variability in human immune system responsiveness as a way to gain a better understanding of genetic susceptibility to vaccine-based adverse events.

Communication

The committee recommends that research be supported to conduct investigations that would deepen and expand the knowledge available from existing studies and more effectively organize what is currently known from these and future projects.

Appendix B
Public Meeting Agenda
February 9, 2004

Immunization Safety Review
Vaccines and Autism

National Academy of Sciences Building
Auditorium, 2100 C Street, NW
Washington, DC

8:00 – 8:15 am   **Welcome and Opening Remarks**
Marie McCormick, M.D., Sc.D., Committee Chair

8:15 – 8:30 am   **Congressional Speakers**
Congressman Dave Weldon,
U.S. House of Representatives

8:30 – 9:30 am   **Etiologic Factors and Pathogenesis of Autism:**
Evidence from Clinical Studies and Animal Models
Mady Hornig, M.D., Associate Professor,
Columbia University Mailman School of Public Health

9:30 – 10:00 am   **Association of Autistic Spectrum Disorder and MMR Vaccine: A Systematic Review of Current Epidemiological Evidence**
Kumanan Wilson, M.D., M.Sc., Division of Clinical Decision Making and Health Care, Toronto General Research Institute, Canada

10:00 – 10:30 am   **Age at First Measles-Mumps-Rubella Vaccination in Children with Autism and School-Matched Control Subjects**
Frank DeStefano, M.D., Centers for Disease Control and Prevention

10:30 – 10:45 am   **Break**

10:45 – 11:15 am   **Exposure to Thimerosal-Containing Vaccines in U.K. Children and Autism**
Dr. Elizabeth Miller, Head, Immunisation Division, Public Health Laboratory Service, Communicable Disease Surveillance Centre, London

11:15 – 11:45 am   **Vaccine Safety Datalink Study: Autism Outcome**
Robert L. Davis, M.D., M.P.H., University of Washington Group Health, Cooperative Departments of Pediatrics Center for Health Studies and Epidemiology

11:45 – 12:15 pm   **Study of the Association Between Thimerosal-Containing Vaccine and Autism in Denmark**
Anders Peter Hviid, M.Sc., Department of Epidemiology Research, State Serum Institute, Copenhagen, Denmark

12:15 – 12:45 pm   **Autism and Thimerosal-Containing Vaccines: Analysis of the Vaccine Adverse Events Reporting System (VAERS)**
Mark R. Geier, M.D., Ph.D., President, The Genetic Centers of America
David Geier, President of MedCon

12:45 – 1:45 pm   **Lunch**

1:45 – 2:15 pm   **A Toxicologist's View of Thimerosal and Autism**
H. Vasken Aposhian, Ph.D., Professor, Molecular and Cellular Biology, University of Arizona

2:15 – 2:45 pm   **Relation of Neurotoxic Effects of Thimerosal to Autism**
David Baskin, M.D., Professor of Neurosurgery and Anesthesiology, Baylor College of Medicine

2:45 – 3:15 pm   **Thimerosal Exposure from Vaccines and Ethylmercury Accumulation in Nonhuman Primates**
Dr. Polly Sager, Assistant Director for International Research, National Institute of Allergy and Infectious Diseases

3:15 – 3:30 pm   **Break**

3:30 – 4:00 pm   **Reduced Levels of Mercury in First Baby Haircuts of Autistic Children**
Boyd Haley, Ph.D., Chairman and Professor, Department of Chemistry, University of Kentucky

4:00 – 4:30 pm   **A Case-Control Study of Mercury Burden in Children with Autistic Disorders and Measles Virus Genomic RNA in Cerebrospinal Fluid in Children with Regressive Autism**
Jeff Bradstreet, M.D., FAAFP, Adjunct Professor, Neurosciences, Stetson University, Director of Clinical Programs, International Child Development Resource Center, Florida

4:30 – 5:00 pm   **Autism, Vaccines, and Immune Reactions**
Vijendra K. Singh, Ph.D., Research Associate Professor, Utah State University

5:00 – 5:30 pm   **Public Comment Period**

5:30 pm   **Adjourn**

Appendix C

Thimerosal Content in Licensed Vaccines (Adapted from FDA, 2003, 2004)

TABLE C-1 Mercury Content from Thimerosal in the Routinely
Recommended Pediatric Vaccines[1] in the United States, April 2004

Vaccine	Brand Name	Manufacturer	Hg [µg/dose]
DTaP (Diphtheria and tetanus toxoids and acellular pertussis)	Tripedia Infanrix Daptacel	Aventis Pasteur, Inc. Glaxo-SmithKline Aventis Pasteur, Ltd	≤0.3 0 0
Td[1] (Tetanus and diphtheria toxoids)	None Decavac None None	Aventis Pasteur, Inc. Aventis Pasteur, Inc. Aventis Pasteur, Ltd Mass Public Health	25 ≤ 0.3 0 8.3
DTaP-Hib (Diphtheria and tetanus toxoids with acellular pertussis combined with *Haemophilus influenzae* type b)	TriHIBit[2]	Aventis Pasteur	≤0.3
Hib (*Haemophilus influenzae* type b)	ActHIB/OmniHib HibTITER (Single dose) PedvaxHIB liquid	Aventis Pasteur, SA Wyeth-Lederle Merck	0 0 0
Hib/HepB (*Haemophilus influenzae* type b combined with Hepatitis B)	COMVAX	Merck	0
Hep B (Hepatitis B) *(pediatric formulation)*	Engerix B Recombivax HB	Glaxo-SmithKline Merck	<0.5 0
Influenza	Fluzone[3] Fluzone (Preservative Free)	Aventis Pasteur, Inc. Aventis Pasteur, Inc.	12.5 ≤0.5ug/ 0.25mL dose
Pneumococcal	Prevnar (pneumoconjugate)	Wyeth	0
IPV **(Inactivated polio vaccine)**	IPOL Poliovax	Aventis Pasteur, SA Aventis Pasteur, Ltd.	0 0
MMR **(Measles, mumps, and rubella)**	MMR-II	Merck	0
Varicella	Varivax	Merck	0

[1]Licensed for persons 7 years of age and older.
[2]For use in children 15 to 18 months of age.
[3]Influenza vaccine is recommended for children 6-23 months of age. *MMWR* (2004) 52:1-4;
MMWR (2004) 53:1-3.

TABLE C-2 Mercury Content from Thimerosal in the Currently Licensed Vaccines That Are Recommended for Some Children in the United States, April 2004

Vaccine	Brand Name	Manufacturer	Hg [μg/dose]
DT (Diphtheria and tetanus toxoids)	All Products	Aventis Pasteur, Inc. (single dose)	0.3
		Aventis Pasteur, Inc. (multi-dose)	25
		Aventis Pasteur, Ltd*	25
TT (Tetanus Toxoid)	All Products	Aventis Pasteur, Inc.	25
Pneumococcal Polysaccharide	Pneumovax 23	Merck	0
Hepatitis A	Havrix	Glaxo-SmithKline	0
	Vaqta	Merck	0
Influenza	Fluzone[1]	Aventis Pasteur, Inc.	25
	Fluzone (Preservative free)	Aventis Pasteur, Inc.	≤1 μg/0.5 mL dose or ≤0.5 μg/ 0.25 mL dose
	Fluvirin	Evans	25
	Fluvirin	Evans	<1 μg
Influenza, Live	FluMist	MedImmune	0

*Not available in the United States.
[1]Children under 3 years of age received half of a vaccine dose (0.25 mL or 12.5 μg mercury/dose).

TABLE C-3   Mercury Content from Thimerosal in Other Licensed Vaccines in the United States, April 2004

Vaccine	Brand Name	Manufacturer	Hg [μg/dose]
Anthrax	BioThrax	BioPort Corporation	0
Smallpox	Dryvax	Wyeth	0
BCG*		Organon Tecknika	0
	Mycobax	Aventis Pasteur, Ltd	0
Hepatitis A-Hepatitis B	Twinrix	Glaxo-SmithKline	<1 μg
Hepatitis B	Engerix B *(adult formulation)*	Glaxo-SmithKline	< 0.5
	Recombivax HB *(adult formulation)*	Merck	25
	Recombivax HB *(adult formulation)*	Merck	0
Lyme*	LYMErix	Glaxo-SmithKline	0
Meningococcal[1]	Menomune A, C, AC and A/C/Y/W-135	Aventis Pasteur, Inc. (multidose)	25
		Single dose	0
Rabies	IMOVAX	Aventis Pasteur SA	0
	Rabavert	Chiron Behring	0
Typhoid Fever	Typhim Vi	Aventis Pasteur SA	0
	Vivotif Berna	Berna Biotech, Ltd.	0
Yellow Fever	YF-VAX	Aventis Pasteur, Inc.	0
Japanese Encephalitis Vaccine	JE-VAX	Aventis Pasteur, Inc.	35

*Not available in the United States.
[1]Menomune A/C/Y/W-135, a thimerosal-containing vaccine, is not indicated for infants and children younger than 2 years of age except as short-term protection of infants 3 months and older against Group A. (*Physician's Desk Reference*, 2001).

Appendix D

Chronology of Important Events Regarding Vaccine Safety

Year	Vaccine Licensure	Legislation and/or Policy Statements	IOM Reports on Vaccine Safety
1955	Inactivated poliomyelitis vaccine (IPV) available		
1963	Oral poliomyelitis vaccine (OPV) available, replaces IPV		
	Measles vaccine available		
1967	Mumps vaccine available		
1969	Rubella vaccine available		
1971	Measles-Mumps-Rubella (MMR) vaccine available		
1977		Mumps vaccination recommended	*Evaluation of Poliomyelitis Vaccines*
1979	Current formulation of rubella vaccine available, replaces earlier versions		
1982	Plasma-derived hepatitis B vaccine available		

Year	Vaccine Licensure	Legislation and/or Policy Statements	IOM Reports on Vaccine Safety
1985	Hib vaccine licensed for children >15 months		
1986		Congress passes P.L. 99-660, the National Childhood Vaccine Injury Act (introduced in 1984) calls for: • est. of NVPO • est. of NVAC • est. of VICP • est. of ACCV IOM review of (1) pertussis and rubella, (2) routine child vaccines	
1988			*Evaluation of Poliomyelitis Vaccine Policy Options*
1990	Two Hib conjugate vaccines licensed for use beginning at 2 months		
1991	Acellular pertussis component licensed for the 4th and 5th doses of the 5-part DTP series in ACEL-IMUNE	Hepatitis B recommended by ACIP for addition to childhood immunization schedule ACIP recommends Hib be added to childhood immunization schedule	*Adverse Effects of Pertussis and Rubella Vaccines*
1992	Acellular pertussis component licensed for the 4th and 5th doses of the 5-part DTP series in Tripedia	Hepatitis B vaccine: Added universal vaccination for all infants, high-risk adolescents (e.g., IV drug users, persons with multiple sex partners)	
1993	Combined DTP and Hib vaccine (Tetramune) licensed		

Year	Vaccine Licensure	Legislation and/or Policy Statements	IOM Reports on Vaccine Safety
1994			*Adverse Events Associated with Childhood Vaccines: Evidence Bearing on Causality*
			DPT and Chronic Nervous System Dysfunction: A New Analysis
1995	Varicella virus vaccine available (Varivax)		
1996	DTaP vaccine licensed for first three doses given in infancy (Tripedia and ACEL-IMUNE were previously licensed for only the 4th and 5th doses).	ACIP recommends using IPV for the first 2 polio vaccinations, followed by OPV for remaining doses. Intended to be a transitional schedule for 3–5 years until an all-IPV series is available	*Options for Poliomyelitis Vaccinations in the United States: Workshop Summary*
		ACIP recommends children 12 months to 12 years receive Varicella vaccine	
1997	Additional DTaP vaccine (Infanrix) licensed for first 4 doses of 5-part series	ACIP recommends DTaP in place of DTP	*Vaccine Safety Forum: Summary of Two Workshops*
			Risk Communication and Vaccination: Workshop Summary
1998	Additional DTaP vaccine (Certiva) licensed for first 4 doses of 5-part series	ACIP updates MMR recommendation, encouraging use of the combined MMR vaccine	

Year	Vaccine Licensure	Legislation and/or Policy Statements	IOM Reports on Vaccine Safety
1999		ACIP updates varicella vaccine recommendation, requiring immunity for child care and school entry	
		ACIP recommends an all-IPV schedule to begin January 2000 to prevent cases of vaccine-associated paralytic polio	
		AAP and PHS recommend removal of thimerosal from vaccines Also recommended postponement of hepatitis B vaccine from birth to 2-6 months for infants of hepatitis B surface antigen-negative mothers	
	Additional supply of thimerosal-free hepatitis B vaccine made available	*MMWR* notifies readers of the availability of a thimerosal-free hepatitis B vaccine, enabling the resumption of the birth dose	
2000	Pneumococcal vaccine for infants and young children licensed (Prevnar)	ACIP recommends pneumococcal vaccination for all children 2-23 months, and at-risk children 24-59 months (e.g., immunocompromised)	
2001		October: ACIP drafts statement expressing a preference for use of thimerosal-free DTaP, Hib, and Hep B vaccines by March 2002	*Immunization Safety Review: Measles-Mumps-Rubella Vaccine and Autism* *Immunization Safety Review: Thimerosal-Containing Vaccines and Neurodevelopmental Disorders*

Year	Vaccine Licensure	Legislation and/or Policy Statements	IOM Reports on Vaccine Safety
2002			*Immunization Safety Review: Multiple Immunizations and Immune Dysfunction*
			Immunization Safety Review: Hepatitis B Vaccine and Demyelinating Neurological Disorders
			Immunization Safety Review: SV40 Contamination of Polio Vaccine and Cancer
2003	Live attenuated intranasal influenza vaccine approved for use in the United States in healthy individuals aged 5-49 years old (FluMist)	ACIP recommends that children 6 to 23 months of age be vaccinated annually against influenza beginning in the 2004-2005 influenza season	*Immunization Safety Review: Hepatitis B Vaccine and Demyelinating Neurological Disorders*
			Immunization Safety Review: SV40 Contamination of Polio Vaccine and Cancer
			Immunization Safety Review: Vaccinations and Sudden Unexpected Death in Infancy
2004			*Immunization Safety Review: Influenza Vaccines and Neurological Complications*

Appendix E

Summary of Public Submissions

Since the announcement of the topic of this report, the committee has received many submissions from the public via mail, email, and fax, all of which were reviewed by the committee to help inform their conclusions and recommendations of this report. A list of all literature and submissions reviewed by the committee can be found on the projects website at www.iom.edu/imsafety.

The unpublished data reviewed by the committee and cited in this report are available—in the form in which they were reviewed—through the public access files of the National Academies. Information about the public access files can be obtained at 202-334-3543 or www.national-academies.org/publicaccess.

The committee is thankful to all those who submitted information. Below is a partial list (as of May 1, 2004) of documents received from the public, broken down into six categories.

1) SCIENTIFIC ARTICLES

The committee received recommendations of published articles to review and often hard copies as well. These were too numerous to list here, but a complete list can be viewed at the Public Access Office (contact information listed above). The committee and IOM staff also did an extensive literature review to find all relevant materials. The following people submitted articles, abstracts, and article recommendations to the committee:

- Sallie Bernard (SafeMinds)
- Jeff Bradstreet (International Child Development Resource Center)

- Amy Carson, Angela Medlin, Karey Williams (Moms Against Mercury)
- Deborah Darnley
- Richard C. Deth (professor of pharmacology)
- Raymond Gallup (The Autism Autoimmunity Project)
- David A. Geier (President, MedCon, Inc.)
- Mark R. Geier (President, The Genetic Centers of America)
- Joseph R. Herr
- Julio Licinio (Nature Publishing Group)
- Becky Nelson
- Lyn Redwood (SafeMinds)
- Daniel J. Thomasch (Orrick)
- Lauren Underwood (Developmental Delay Consultant, Inc.)
- American Autism Association

2) PERSONAL STATEMENTS

The committee received many accounts from parents that described their situation and their child or family member with autism, sometimes with medical histories and/or medical documents enclosed. The committee also received personal statements on the topic of autism and vaccines in general from the following people:

- American Autism Association; Sponsored by parents of children with autism. We want you to know the truth (folder containing articles, papers, scientific journal articles, and letters).
- Teresa A. Anderson (Immunization Action Coalition), 2004. Vaccines and Autism.
- Trish Berger, 2004. Relationship of MMR Vaccine to Autistic Spectrum.
- James and Kathy Blanco, 2004. Children Left Behind.
- Kathy Blanco, 2004. Autism Increase
- Kathy Blanco, 2004. Read at your meeting today, urgent!
- Robert Chen, 2004. IOM—Vaccines and Autism meeting on 2/9/04
- Alan Clark, 2004.
- Deborah Darnley, 2004. *Medical records and personal statement*
- Anne Ferreira, 2004. Immunization Safety Review Committee Meeting 9: Vaccines and Autism
- Maurice Frank, 2004. Media freedom implications of autism vaccine dangers
- Raymond Gallup, 2004. IOM—Vaccines and Autism
- Michelle Gibson, 2004. Autism nine feedback
- Audrey Hamilton, 2004. Autism-vaccines
- Diane Litt, 2004. MMR Vaccine and autism
- Donald Meserlian, 2004. VOSI Input for Immunization Safety Review: Vaccines and Autism...Meeting nine

- Marjorie H. Monteleon (Maine DEP Dental Mercury Workgroup), 2004. Reference to the Immunization Safety review Committee Meeting 2/9/04.
- National Autism Association: Folder with stories from the families of children with autism (sponsored by individual parents). We want you to know the truth...
- Sylvia Nichols, 2004. Autism and Vaccinations.
- Clarence W. Tiske, 2004. Autism meeting nine, sedation thimerosal.
- Lauren Underwood, 2004. Immunization Safety Review.
- Linda Weinmaster, 2004. IOM vaccines and autism public comment.
- American Autism Assocation; Sponsored by parents of autistic children.

The committee also received several submissions from the public stating potential theories of how vaccines/thimerosal injure children/adults together with unpublished background information and critiques of data.

- Catherine Boyle, 2004. Immunization Safety Review—vaccines and autism: what about mitochondrial disease underlying autism?
- Amy Carson, Angela Medlin, Karey Williams (Moms Against Mercury), 2004. Removal of all Mercury Products in Vaccines.
- Enayati, A. New Autism Data: Slight Decrease May Reflect Mercury Removal from Vaccines (Schafer Autism Report).
- M.R. Geier, D.A. Geier. 2004. Important additional considerations for the IOM committee on thimerosal.
- M.R. Geier, D.A. Geier. 2004. New Important Additional Considerations for the IOM committee on Thimerosal II and III.
- M.R. Geier, D.A. Geier. 2004. VAERS Database Raw Data for Independent Methodology Verification.
- M.R. Geier, D.A. Geier. 2004. VSD Raw Data: Thimerosal and Autism.
- Elizabeth Mumper (Advocates for Children, Ltd.), 2004. *Letter.*
- J.D. Nordin, M. Goodman, D.M. Smeltzer, E.P. Ehlinger, K. Kephart. 2004. Commentary on data presented by the Geiers at the thimerosal meeting.
- Lyn Redwood (SafeMinds), 2004. IOM 2-04 RhoD comments.
- Lyn Redwood (SafeMinds), 2004. IOM 5-04 Primate Study comments.
- Lyn Redwood (SafeMinds). VSD Comments to IOM 02-16-04.
- Glen F. Rall (Fox Chase Cancer Center), 2004. *Letter.*

3) UNPUBLISHED PAPERS

The committee received many unpublished papers to supplement published articles. These include:

- S. Bernard (SafeMinds), 2004. Analysis of the Autism Registry Data Base in Response to the Hviid et al. Paper on Thimerosal in *JAMA* (October, 2003).

- S. Bernard (SafeMinds), 2003. Analysis and Critique of the CDC's Handling of the Thimerosal Exposure Assessment Based on Vaccine Safety Datalink (VSD) information.
- S. Bernard (SafeMinds), 2004. "VSD Thimerosal Analysis of June 2000" Background Information on this Document by SafeMinds.
- Teresa Binstock (researcher), 2004. Increased susceptibility to adverse effects from vaccinations.
- M. Blaxill, L. Redwood, S. Bernard (submitted by: SafeMinds). Thimerosal and Autism? A plausible hypothesis that should not be dismissed. A response to: K.B. Nelson and M.L. Bauman. (2003) Thimerosal and Autism? *Pediatrics* 111(3):674-9.
- J. Bradstreet, 2004. Biological Evidence of Significant Vaccine Related Side-effects Resulting in Neurodevelopmental Disorders.
- J. Bradstreet. 2004. Is There a Nexus for MMR and Mercury Issues in Autism Spectrum Disorders.
- R. Deth, 2004. Molecular Basis of the Link Between Thimerosal and Autism.
- M. Geier and D. Geier, 2004. From Epidemiology, Clinical Medicine, Molecular Biology, and Atoms, to Politics: A Review of the Relationship between Thimerosal and Autism.
- E.H. Granai, 2004. Are Some Cases of Autism the Result of a Persistent, Attenuated Rubella Infection in the Mother?
- E.H. Granai, 2004. The Phenomenon of a Concentration of Autistic Children's Births in the Months of March and August.
- B. Haley, 2004. Biomedical Aspects of Thimerosal Exposure.
- S.J. James, 2004. Impaired transsulfuration and oxidative stress in autistic children: Improvement with targeted nutritional intervention (submitted by J. Bradstreet).
- V. Singh, 2004. Autism, Vaccines, and Immune Reactions.

4) TRANSCRIPTS AND CONGRESSIONAL RECORDS

- Congressional Record—Extension of Remarks. May 20, 3003. Mercury in Medicine Report. Hon. Dan Burton of Indiana, In the House of Representatives (submitted by Mark and David Geier).
- Dan Burton. May 2003. Mercury in Medicine; Taking Unnecessary Risks. (A report Prepared by the Staff of the Subcommittee on Human Rights and Wellness, Committee on Government Reform, United States House of Representatives) (submitted by Mark and David Geier).
- Dan Burton (Chairman): Opening statement; "FACA: Conflicts of Interest and Vaccine Development: Preserving the Integrity of the Process. June 15, 2000. Washington, DC. (submitted by R. Gallup, The Autism Autoimmunity Project).

- Simpsonwood Transcript. *Scientific Review of Vaccine Safety Datalink Information, June 7-8, 2000.* Simpsonwood Retreat Center, Norcross, GA (submitted by M. and D. Geier).
- Transcript from the High Court of Justice hearing in the matter of MMR/MR vaccine litigation, Case Management Conference (submitted by D. Salisbury).
- Transcript—U.S. House of Representatives, Government Reform Committee holds a hearing on the status of the research into vaccine safety and autism. 6/19/02 (submitted by J. Bradstreet).

5) QUESTIONS TO CONSIDER

Several people emailed questions for the committee to consider while reviewing the research regarding autism, thimerosal, MMR, and mercury. They included:

- Raymond Gallup, 2004. Question???-February 9, 2004 meeting-autism and vaccines.
- Tonya Harbison, 2004. Autism.
- Michelle Mitchell, 2004. Topics for discussion in vaccine/autism meetings.

6) NEWS ARTICLES

The committee also received news articles, including those listed below.

- Assessing the Role of Mercury in Autism. 2002. By: Boyd E. Haley. *Mothering Magazine* (submitted by Moms Against Mercury).
- Autism in a Needle? The toxic tale of vaccinations and mercury poisoning (11/11/03) By: Annette Fuentes (submitted by M. and D. Geier).
- Methylmercury Toxicology Probed. By: Louisa Wray Dalton (submitted by J. Bradstreet).
- New Research Suggests Link Between Vaccine Ingredients and Autism, ADHD (submitted by Becky Nelson).
- The Irresponsible Media Coverage of the Institute of Medicine Meeting on Autism and Vaccines. By: Sandy Mintz, RFD Columnist (submitted by Philip Rudnick, West Chester University of Pennsylvania).
- Vaccine and Autism (12/29/03) and Autism and Vaccines (2/9/04) (submitted by Deborah Wexler, Immunization Action Coalition).
- Water in D.C. Exceeds the EPA Lead Limit; Random Tests Last Summer Found Levels in 4,000 Homes Throughout City. 1/31/04. By: D. Nakamura (submitted by J. Bradstreet).

Appendix F

Acronyms

ADD – attention deficit disorder
ADHD – attention deficit hyperactivity disorder
ADI – Autism Diagnostic Interview
ADOS-G – Autism Diagnostic Observation Schedule-G
APA – American Psychiatric Association
ASD – autistic spectrum disorder
ATSDR – Agency for Toxic Substance and Disease Registry

BSS –Biologic Surveillance Summaries

CDC – Centers for Disease Control and Prevention
CDD – childhood disintegrative disorder
CI – confidence interval
CISA – Clinical Immunization Safety Assessment
CMI – cell-mediated immunity
CNS – central nervous system
ConA – concanavalin A
COPUS – Committee on the Public Understanding of Science

DNA – deoxyribonucleic acid
DOE – U.S. Department of Education
DSM-IV – Diagnostic and Statistical Manual of Mental Disorders—Fourth
    Edition
DT – diphtheria-tetanus vaccine

DTaP – diphtheria-tetanus and acellular pertussis vaccine
DTaPHib – diphtheria-tetanus and acellular pertussis-*Haemophilus influenzae*
   B vaccine
DTP – diphtheria-tetanus and pertussis vaccine
DTwP – diphtheria-tetanus and whole-cell pertussis vaccine
DTwPHIB – diphtheria-tetanus and whole-cell pertussis-*H. influenzae* B
   vaccine

ED – U.S. Department of Education
EPA – U.S. Environmental Protection Agency
EtHg – ethyl mercury

FDA – U.S. Food and Drug Administration

GABHS – group A beta-hemolytic streptococcal
GI – gastrointestinal
GPRD – General Practice Research Database

HBV – hepatitis B virus
Hg – mercury
Hib – *H. influenzae* type b vaccine
HMO – health maintenance organization
HVR-3 – third hypervariable region

IAVG – Interagency Vaccine Group
IBD – inflammatory bowel disease
ICD-10 – International Classification of Diseases, Tenth Revision
IDEA – Individuals with Disabilities Education Act
IGF-1 – insulin-like growth factor 1
IOM – Institute of Medicine
IPV – inactivated polio vaccine
IQ – intelligence quotient score

LBW – low birth weight
LEAD – Leadership Education and Advocacy Development
LLDB – large-linked database
LPS – lipopolysaccharide

MADDSP – Metropolitan Atlanta Disabilities Surveillance Program
MBP – myelin basic protein
MECP2 – methyl-CpG-binding protein 2
MFS –Maudsley Family Study
MHC – Maudsley Hospital Clinic; major histocompatibility complex

MMR – measles-mumps-rubella
MRI – magnetic resonance imaging
mRNA – messenger RNA (messenger ribonucleic acid)
MS – methionine synthase; multiple sclerosis
MT – metallothionein

NBCC – National Breast Cancer Coalition
NBH – National Board of Health
NDD – neurodevelopmental delay
NIH – National Institutes of Health

OD – odds ratio
OPV – oral polio vaccine

PANDAS – pediatric autoimmune neuropsychiatric disorder associated with streptococcal infection
PDD – pervasive developmental disorder
PDD-NOS – pervasive developmental disorder—not otherwise specified
PHA – phytohemagluttinin
PHS – U.S. Public Health Service

RICHS – Regional Interactive Child Health Computing System
RR – risk ratio

SISA – Simple Interactive Statistical Analysis
SSPE – subacute sclerosing panencephalitis

TCV – thimerosal-containing vaccine
TFV – thimerosal-free vaccines

UK – United Kingdom
USPHS – United States Public Health Service

VAERS – Vaccine Adverse Event Reporting System
VICP – Vaccine Injury Compensation Program
VSD – Vaccine Safety Datalink

WHO – World Health Organization
wP – whole-cell pertussis